Why We Never Give Up Our Need for a Perfect Mother

Why We Never Give Up Our Need for a Perfect Mother

◆

Trapped at Home
by
Anxiety & Panic?

Anne Hart,
M.A. Behavioral Science Journalist

ASJA Press
New York Lincoln Shanghai

Why We Never Give Up Our Need for a Perfect Mother
Trapped at Home by Anxiety & Panic?

Copyright © 2007 by Anne Hart

ASJA Press
an imprint of iUniverse, Inc.

iUniverse books may be ordered through booksellers or by contacting:

iUniverse
2021 Pine Lake Road, Suite 100
Lincoln, NE 68512
www.iuniverse.com
1-800-Authors (1-800-288-4677)

ISBN-13: 978-0-595-43402-2
ISBN-10: 0-595-43402-9

Printed in the United States of America

Contents

1

The 5-HTT Gene

How limited are future career plans when you are trapped at home for many years with agoraphobia—the fear of panicking in unfamiliar spaces? Research at the Stoneybrook University in New York revealed that if you inherit a short version of the gene called 5-HTT, you're more likely to be predisposed to experiencing anxiety and fear or to become depressed.

Other studies reveal that you also may be sensitive to carbon dioxide in the air, feeling panicky when the there's 5 percent carbon dioxide in the air. For people without a genetic sensitivity, the air in your environment would have to reach seven percent carbon dioxide before you'd feel anxious.

If you're chronically anxious, have panic disorder or have advanced to agoraphobia, and are afraid of leaving your home or other familiar surroundings, if you can't drive, ride in a bus without getting a white-out, or walk more than a few feet from your home without anxiety causing you to return home.... you may not even feel depressed or be aware of any other feeling but a physical sense of dread, trembling, or numbness in your elbow.

You may panic, feel dizzy, become short of breath, hyperventilate, and go through the fight or flight syndrome. You may have adverse reactions to stress, medicines, anesthesia, or foods. You could become allergic or sensitive to loud sound effects in movie theaters, have a fear of bus travel beyond a certain point, or have white-outs while traveling, perhaps developing more frequent migraines.

You crave healing sounds in music that makes you feel relaxed. Perhaps you are experiencing post traumatic stress disorder. If you don't have agoraphobia, perhaps it is sociophobia that keeps you away from opportunities to meet people and make friends. Or your stress may be from a physical condition that worsens when you talk on the phone or meet new people and have to speak in public. Or your panic may increase when you are in a group and fear that you're being singled out, judged, or discriminated against.

Sometimes you develop an increasing sensitivity to dental anesthetics. For example, you react immediately with a panic attack when given a dental injection, but can be calm when the same minor dental work, such as a deep cleaning on one tooth, is done without anesthesia.

Why do you feel anxious, get panic attacks, or become homebound for decades with agoraphobia? Hyperactivity in the brain's fear center due to the fact that you've inherited a short instead of a long 5-HTT gene could be the cause. The brain's fear center is connected to the amygdala and hippocampus.

Okay, you have a short 5-HTT gene. Maybe you can't travel without become anxious, stressed, or panicked. Maybe you get headaches from travel or have a low stress level. Maybe you panic when you laugh or are in any way emotionally stimulated by sound, touch, sight, scent, or experience.

You may not be able to sit in a movie theater or view a play without feeling anxious from the loud sound effects or the flashing lights. You look for calming experiences. The problem is you have electrical activity in your brain.

The electrical activity is in motion all the time, even when nothing should cause fear—such as when you laugh or make love. You overreact to anything that stimulates that electrical center in your brain's fear center. It doesn't have to be anything that would cause fear to people who have inherited a long copy of the 5-HTT gene.

The world is divided between calm people with a long 5-HTT gene and anxious individuals with a short 5-HTT gene. People with a short 5-HTT gene live with constant electrical activity in their brain's fear center.

You may feel either anxiety or depression if you have a short 5-HTT gene. Look up the article reporting a study that links depression to an overactive fear center in the brain titled, *"Bound for Gloom and Doom,"* Proceedings of the National Academy or Sciences, October 11, 2006. You can find this online at *ScienceNOW Daily News.* Online, check out *ScienceNOW's* search engine at: http://sciencenow.sciencemag.org/cgi/search?searchtype= article&andorexacttitle=or&fulltext=bound+for+gloom+and+doom.

If left untreated, agoraphobia can burn itself out with moderate exercise, but it may take years. You need to study how your genes react to various treatments so that you don't become dependent upon the treatment and not find the cause.

If your problem is post partum anxiety or menopause, and you're concerned about hormonal imbalances on top of genetic predisposition, such as a short 5-HTT gene or defects in your autonomic nervous system inherited at birth compounded by your environment and trauma from physical, emotional, or environmental stress, or even a slight head injury years ago, work on the physiological, nutritional, and genetic causes of what is keeping you bound to your home.

What worked for may be similar or very different from what will work for you. Be sure to find out how your genes react to the buildup of certain vitamins or minerals from food supplements.

Are certain B complex vitamins you take over-stimulating your thyroid? Know your body type, metabolism, and genetic predispositions. Find out how fast or slow your body builds up and metabolizes vitamins, foods, and supplements in ways that might build up in your body to over stimulate glands or organs. Are there toxic substances in the water you're drinking?

Are you using a water distiller that takes out all the magnesium and calcium, and you aren't replacing those minerals in your food supplements so your body can function properly? What trace minerals are you taking?

Who else in your family had anxiety problems, migraines, or other inherited issues? Did a parent smoke, drink too much caffeine or alcohol, or take any medicines or supplements during pregnancy that might have influenced your autonomic nervous system's response to stress or other perceived changes?

When you eat fruit or sugary foods, is there a rush of insulin and adrenalin that makes you tremble with anxiety? Are the sugars in your diet worsening chronic gum disease by keeping your blood glucose level too high? Anaerobic bacteria under the gums thrive on excess sugar and yeast in your blood. Have you looked at your reactions to food that is a combination of protein and good oils such as extra virgin olive oil and Omega 3 fish oils?

Have you discussed with your health professional whether certain foods "hit you like a bomb" and cause anxiety or other symptoms of blood sugar changes?

Agoraphobia has a female-to-male ratio of 2-3:1. Social phobia is more common in females, but more males ask for treatment due to the social pressures on men to earn an income throughout adult life. Talk with health professionals that specialize in these symptoms. Is it metabolic syndrome for you or something else? Do you have the short 5-HTT gene? Or is another part of your body giving you an important message to heed? Find out how your genes process what enters your body and how your genes and brain electro-chemistry react to stress. Stress is rapid change. Does food hit you like a bomb?

What Helped My Own Hyperinsulinism and Metabolic Syndrome

What worked for me may not work for you because your metabolic system is different from mine. You need to tailor your foods and treatments to your own genes and work with health professionals that look at the whole person, and not solely the one symptom. Between 1965 and early 1972 I was housebound with agoraphobia and panic disorder. It began after the birth of my first and second children in March 1965 and in November 1966. It resumed in 1981 to 1985 and from 1999 until 2004 when I started a better nutrition program without eating the chocolate I craved, sugary desserts, and shell fish.

Each body type has different nutritional variations just as you have different genes that can be switched on and off by various methods. My metabolic syndrome and agoraphobia with panic disorder, my sensitivities to carbon dioxide in the air, to dental anesthetics, and to a variety of foods and scents will be different than yours.

What set off anxiety experiences or panic attacks in me or what caused my belly to go convex will be different that what sets off your physical reactions or experiences. Sugar and too much salt, too many dairy products and too little greens were not good for my health. You are different. Keep in mind that your genes influence how food affects your body. What environmental sounds, scents, or experiences affect your panic level?

By switching to vanilla instead of chocolate desserts, and a largely vegetarian Mediterranean and Japanese diet (seaweed, salmon, whole grains, green vegetables, no caffeine, and decaf green tea with lemongrass or herb tea with blueberry leaf), I am now able to travel by bus and walk for a half hour near my home. Caffeine and other foods were wreaking havoc causing adverse reactions as well as most dental anesthetics.

More than two million people in the United States suffer from this incapacitating anxiety, a panic state, when traveling away from their homes. It's a fear that wells up when under even the slightest stress or in an unfamiliar situation.

When traditional medicine failed to help, a friend sent me a book on Yoga exercises and meditation. I practiced the positions with determination to help myself.

In addition to the approximately 28 Yoga postures, I used music therapy, calming ethnic music of strings, flutes, and slow drums at 60 beats per minute to bring down my naturally high adrenaline state. I also changed my diet to vegetarian, but medium-protein, cutting out all white sugar and salted foods, all caffeine and chocolate.

I added raw vegetables and cut out certain starches in high amounts such as cooked potatoes and loads of cooked rice and substituted tofu, protein powder, and grapefruit pectin powder, two scoops per day.

A fish and fruit diet also worked wonders and is helpful for those not strict vegetarians. I was willing to try cooked fresh cold water fish like baked salmon in lemon juice because it's helpful to those with genetic-based hyperinsulinism and genetically high blood pressure.

My monthly estrogen migraines also grew less painful as a result. The vitamins I took were Vitamin E with 100 mg. of Selenium, Vitamin C, and beta carotene, and the usual B complex vitamins found in health food stores in normal amounts fewer than 100 mg. I also took magnesium 400 and calcium 600 to 1000 mgs.

At the time I was 25 years old. I'm in my late sixties now. I couldn't exercise much with agoraphobia because exercise increased the lactic acid in my body. Lactic acid creates panic attacks in persons prone to panic disorder. Exercising caused exercise asthma, hyperventilation syndrome, and panic attacks.

During pregnancy, the estrogen and progesterone levels increase dramatically in a woman's body. A pregnant woman has 200 times as much estrogen in her body than before or after pregnancy. After childbirth, that estrogen and progesterone level drops suddenly. For me, the result was panic attacks with agoraphobia and hyperventilation syndrome.

One way for me to get rid of my fear of leaving the house and the panic attacks was to get pregnant again. By the third month of pregnancy I'd feel incredibly calm again. But I couldn't do that forever, especially, not when my husband divorced me after the second child.

Yoga was my next resort. Yoga required stretching instead of the usual exercise movement that would increase my already hyper state of adrenaline and insulin in my blood. In addition, I had low blood sugar (hypoglycemia)and too much insulin as I previously mentioned—(genetic hyperinsulinism). Too much insulin from too many fast burning carbohydrates grew me a protruding belly that didn't look great on my 112 pound five feet four body. My fasting blood glucose of 86 would drop to 60 when I drank two tablespoons of honey in lemon water during a glucose tolerance test.

For seven years I was totally housebound and suffered dozens of panic attacks a day some days. Other days I'd only have chronic anxiety for the entire day, and panic when I had to sit in my graduate school classroom. At the time I was an evening school graduate student in genetic and medical anthropology and science journalism. I'd tried every exercise from aerobics to belly dancing.

Yoga was the only movement that relaxed me without giving me exercise asthma and the tremors. The stretching of my muscles removed the lactic acid from my body in the same way that a runner stretches a leg against a tree to cool down and remove the lactic acid that builds up in the body during exercise. It was the build up of lactic acid causing me to shake with the tremors and go into a panic attack upon exercise.

Persons who are biologically prone to agoraphobia and panic under the slightest stress normally are born with shy, over-aroused dominant introverted feeling) nervous systems. They often secrete a high level of catecholamines. Their adrenaline level is frequently at a higher base level than in the average or naturally calm person. They secrete more insulin into their blood that people who are literally immune from anxiety attacks.

Sometimes the left hemisphere of the brain (high verbal intelligence) begins to fire at a different rate, faster or slower, than the right hemisphere (visual art and emotion). When the two hemispheres get out of sync, panic and shaking could occur at any time of the night or day, when you laugh or sleep, walk through the street or sit in a chair.

Stretching from the Yoga positions calmed me so that I could relax and enjoy the day's events. I'd been a person with an avoidant/dependent personality type. I withdrew from direct people contact and became a recluse in order to stop being a "hot reactor."

An 'invisible' hot reactor reacts to the slightest stress not by outward anger, but inwardly and silently, by a dramatically increased blood pressure, pulse rate, and sudden, gripping fear to people and slight mental stress, even though there is no facial expression change or bodily motion to show what's narrowing or calcifying from sugar (and insulin's overabundance to sugar) on the inside.

All I ended up with was the protruding pot belly of hyperinsulinism—on the thin, small-boned frame of a 120 pound, medium-height woman. It's also called metabolic disease. In my situation, it combined with agoraphobic, panic disorder, chronic anxiety and sociophobia—fear of people, loud sounds, and ringing telephones. Outwardly, emotion is introverted, so nobody can see what you're feeling on the inside.

Sometimes closet extroverts forced to act like introverts to please introverted family members in power can help to push a genetically prone person into panic disorder. Usually, some physical stress does it, such as childbirth, surgery, or even getting married or a first job and moving out of the family.

You can also get panic disorder from watching your mother being battered and not being able to help at a young age, or getting frightened by a parent. It signifies a sense of loss and fear of losing your health, and it prevents you from traveling, or in my case, of learning to drive. I never did learn to drive, but by choice. Why? I went from a low-income housewife (homemaker) to a low-income senior citizen.

Why learn to drive when I did not own a car or have the income to pay for a car, let alone the yearly insurance. I couldn't even become a member of a house of worship because it would cost money each month or annually, and with no income, food, clothing, and a bus pass became priorities. Luckily, I don't have to pay rent at this time. I know too well what it feels like to be homeless. Again, being homeless at the age of 28 felt very different from what it would feel like now as I move closer to the age 70 mark when the most important indicator of integrity in addition to health is being independent and in your own home.

I had to change my diet to healing foods that would not further stimulate my thyroid, as sugar and simple carbohydrates were doing when they quickly turned to sugar as soon as they reached my bloodstream. Examples were fruit juice, white rice, bran muffins, and bagels.

As a biological introvert, sensitive to people's actions, noise, intrusions, and words, my whole body would over react to any stress in my environment, until I had to back off and become housebound. I couldn't work at any job that brought me into contact with people directly.

The phone would ring and my pulse and pressure would hit the ceiling. I couldn't sit in cinema theaters as the sounds effects were so loud that they caused panic attacks. The loud effects overwhelmed my nervous system and caused panic tremors that subsided when the film or loud music had finished. Gentle string and harp music calmed me, especially Baroque music of the 17th century and new age meditation music.

I didn't dare answer the phone or I'd go into hyperventilation syndrome and start breathing too fast in terror at the voice on the other end. I was expending a ton of energy in response to an ounce of provocation. I was afraid of everything that could elicit a physiological response in me. Bellydance music, if not loud, created a feeling of well-being and prayer.

To counteract my weak calming branch, the more I stretched with Yoga exercises, the cooler and calmer I became. I noticed that at the height of my panic attack, I'd go into the Yoga positions and stretch my muscles. The result was a sudden sense of calm. Qi Gong and Tai Chi helped improve my balance. I've always had problems keeping my balance, even when young, during the post-partum phase when agoraphobia and panic disorder hit hard, keeping me housebound exactly at the moment my then wife-beating husband (now many decades deceased) had filed for divorce, taking all the money in the bank account, removing the children to a foreign country, selling the house, and leaving me homeless and penniless.

Imagine what it feels like to be homeless and housebound with agoraphobia, panic disorder, and hyperinsulinism/metabolic syndrome, and chronic anxiety at the same moment your physically abusive husband walks out, leaving the coun-

try, even his mistress giving you the finger, taking all the children and money …
and you have no relatives of your own family to offer a hand. (He later also left
his mistress when he left the country.) That's what happened to me.

Even when without more than a few cents left on the table, I determined that
I would exercise agoraphobia away, back then in the mid 1960s, when I was only
in my late twenties. Little did I know then that my son would grow up and
become a physician specializing in neuroradiology, and my daughter (a language
scholar) would marry a physician who works with these types of issues in the field
of internal medicine.

What about the anxiety that kept me from going more than a few feet from
my home? I hadn't realized that the amounts of vitamin B complex I took stimulated my large, fast thyroid so much that the anxiety increased even more.

What I hadn't realized is that vitamin B (complex) stimulates the thyroid. In
my body, my particular genes allowed the vitamin to over stimulate my thyroid
because of my sensitivity to various types of vitamin B.

That's why it's important to find out how your genes turn on and off in reaction to food and food supplements and how these vitamins affect other parts of
your body. It's all about how your genes respond to food, medicine, or environment.

When I walked for a half hour or more a day in small, 10 minute walking sessions, the anxiety would fade. A feeling of sending out waves of love to my worst
enemy took over my body and mind. My dominant introverted feeling personality type emphasized values. I asked myself: Is this issue worth weakening my
heart's pacemaker by an adrenaline bath? The answer was always, of course not.
For me, music became a healing tone. The type of music affected my brain's fear
or calming center and healed my body to the point of a feeling of well-being
instead of anxiety.

Harp music, calming sting music, and even slow, new age music relaxed me.
Belly dance music and music of India allowed me to stretch and do my Tai-Chi
exercises to the music as well as Yoga-type stretches. From there, I moved to
high-energy bellydancing alone in my room, stretching out my arms in a type of
dance-prayer-tai-chi and yoga stretch and moving my arms and shoulders or feet
in a folk or tribal dance. When done in short spans, not long, exhausting hip-
drops, the exercise did calm me, and a feeling of well-being arose along with stress
reduction. Nutrition played a part. I had to balance my magnesium and calcium
to feel relaxed.

Now, my body had to understand that feeling value at the molecular level as
well. The best and healthiest answers came when I asked a value question, is it

worth it? Worth it meant was the solution, need, benefit, or answer worth it to my health in the long run.

Yoga was the best event in my writing life and in providing a link or bridge to learning to relax by stretching until calm. Listening to calming music or chanting also was a relaxing experience during a panic episode.

The calming, ethnic or meditative new age music such as Indian music relaxed me. My whole body would physiologically react to the beat of the music. The slow beats, precisely music of 60 beats per minute brought me down to a relaxed normal feeling.

Music distracted my brain from firing off anxiety neurons. The right hemisphere of my brain was shooting off energy from neurons a lot faster that the left hemisphere of my brain when the both hemispheres should have been working together in balance at more or less the same rate. This was another cause of my chronic anxiety, panic attacks, and ultimately being housebound with agoraphobia (literally, fear of the outdoors). I turned to Ayurvedic medical books for kind solace. Yoga helped the most along with Qi Gong, a form of Tai Chi for health and balance.

What I was really afraid of was not the marketplace, or outdoors (agora in Greek), but my body's panic reaction to stress. I perceived stress as threatening so fast that my logical side didn't have time to calm myself down. I had a weak calming branch.

Again Yoga came to the rescue. How Yoga worked specifically was by the actual stretching of the muscles. When muscles stretch they cool down the panic by changing the posture. The stretching removed the adrenaline, lactic acid, and insulin from the muscles, and the muscles stopped shaking.

My breathing grew slower as I stretched and went through the basic postures. My monthly migraines eased. Meditation became easier. Finally, I could relax after a good, but gentle Yoga stretch. What's your body type? Different body types metabolize nutrients according to their own physiology. There are fast and slow 'metabolizers.' Have yours checked and measured.

Stretching Away the Panic Attacks

To get rid of the panic attack, I'd begin by sitting in a half lotus position. For hyperventilation syndrome, I'd breathe into a brown paper bag to increase the carbon dioxide. However, when I was back to normal, I'd breathe fresh air slowly because carbon dioxide causes sensitive people with panic disorder to have a panic attack from breathing carbon dioxide. Then I'd hold my left foot firmly and place my left foot and heel against my right middle thigh near the knee while stretching my arms downward.

The position of my foot resting against my inner thigh became the most calming stretch position for me. I tried to stretch my arm muscles and the rest of my leg muscles. Then I allowed my forearm to relax and rest against my raised knee. I'd sit for two minutes in this posture. The weight of my forearm gradually lowered my knee. By the time the knee was lowered as far as it needed to go, I was calmed down. Slow deep breathing was very helpful.

Yoga also helped my inner ear problems. I have a damaged left inner ear from the time I was a passenger in the back seat of a car that was rear ended in an accident in 1967.

After the ear injuries healed, I had life long vertigo attacks whenever I was under stress. The stretching and movement of yoga as a series of postures helped me regain my balance.

Eventually my brain compensated for the damaged inner ear, and the vertigo and ear problems lessened, especially by the side bend Yoga exercise. I'd recommend to any person housebound by agoraphobia to check out the values of a Yoga regimen backed up by balanced nutrition, vitamins and minerals, and meditation with music therapy. Of all the therapies I tried, Yoga worked the best.

Now years later, I practice Yoga. It's combined with slow belly dancing and Tai Chi Chuan, meditation, slow beat ethnic, new age, and classical music. I ate soaked over night and then slow, low-heat-cooked whole grains and legumes consumed with fresh and juiced vegetables, and no sugar or excessive salt. Fast dancing only brought on exercise asthma for me. Stretching slowly took it away.

My motto is "stretch your panic away." I'd take this regimen anytime over tranquilizers, addictive drugs with side effects, or antidepressants that do nothing for the panic, but treat the depression that are usually prescribed for agoraphobia with panic disorder. I'm only speaking for myself here.

I didn't feel depressed. I felt scar out of my skin, scared to tremors. The seizure of shaking felt almost like a mild epileptic set of convulsions. Yet, I was always told after seeing dozens of doctors that nothing showed up on tests.

Back then, in the middle sixties, my doctors told me my panic attacks were all in my head, and I was in good health. They automatically gave me a prescription for Miltown or Librium. I didn't take the tranquilizers after hearing other people's sensitivity reactions to the pills. I wanted to try more natural solutions to agoraphobia and panic disorder such as better foods or vitamins and minerals or antioxidants in small amounts. What worked best for me focused on mild exercise, walking in place, then walking outdoors, then Tai Chi, Qi Gong and gentle

Yoga. Finally, bellydancing or tribal dancing alone in my room to relaxing but exotic music that allowed me to stretch and relax.

When I got older and complained of too much adrenaline in my blood, they gave me a prescription for Inderal, a beta blocker to stop adrenalin from hitting my heart's electrical system. Over the years, I'd developed arrythmias which I cured with 150 mg. of selenium, 400 mg of vitamin E, 300 mg. of magnesium, calcium, and the amino acid, a little Taurine (half or quarter of a 500 mg capsule) or Coenzyme Q 10 in a bottle of multiple vitamins.

I never took the pills because I was afraid of the side effects of depression, which I didn't have in the first place. Instead, vitamins, minerals such as 400 mgs of magnesium and an equal amount of calcium with a tiny amount—a half capsule of the amino acid Taurine, helped me feel normal. Omega 3 fish oil helped most along with good nutrition.

I know that having a genetically sensitive to stress system helped me understand why I feel so well working at home where I can have my own flexible work hours. Yoga did help as did my vitamin B complex regimen with (for me only) 800 mgs of folic acid in the B complex capsules and Betaine. These helped me along with Yoga. Everything, in vitamins or minerals, for me, is in moderation. Please do not copy my individual combination of nutrients are for my body type. Make sure you tailor your own foods and nutrients to your own body, genes, and blood type constitution.

I also have AB blood that needs a balance of protein and carbohydrates because I don't have the thin type O blood that can eat a lot of protein, but rather the "vegetarian with some fish, fish oil, olive oil, and sea vegetables" (the omega 3 and 6 oils in balance as fatty acids) 'thicker' blood type, that is found in the healthy diets of Japan and the Mediterranean areas.

Optimism helped the most to walk-off and dance away anxiety. Hope helps. Healing music, exercise, and nutritious eating became my regimen. I preferred Yoga, meditation, serenity, good nutrition, and the vitamins and minerals that keep me calm and reduce my reactions to stress.

For me stretching with Yoga eventually helped my menopausal back-aches, when I went through menopause more than fifteen years ago. Taken with the best nutrition plan that works for me, stretching in Yoga and balancing from Tai Chi Chuan stepping gives me the right kind of weight bearing exercise I need now in my sixth-going-on-seventh decade.

Making my own almond milk and eating frozen blueberries also helped to calm me. Fresh blue berries remove some of the vitamin B from you. Frozen or cooked blueberries don't because the B vitamin removing enzyme is disabled by freezing or cooking. I take a scoop of soy protein to help my bones and arteries. Along with the Yoga and Tai Chi Chuan exercise program or walking as I don't drive, I'm happy and able to write to the best of my ability. Thanks, everyone, and thanks for Yoga.

It's the stretching and relaxation that works for me with world beat music in the background, again keeping to 60 beats per minute when I can find it. I particularly like the music CD, *Sheltering Stones*, by Richard Searles (Earth Dance Music, Sherman Oaks, CA).

Instrumentals with gentle voice sounds as in Mystic Voyage, from the CD Sheltering Stones, is a calming, Celtic work of plucked strings and soft voices that helps me to visualize misty and mystic mornings at Big Sur in California.

Unsweetened products such as unsweetened almond milk has reputation for building bones, (but be sure to find out how your body reacts to taking calcium and magnesium supplements so you get enough, but not too much to trigger other problems) and Yoga is known for stretching and calming.

To counteract my weak calming branch, the more I stretched with Yoga exercises, the cooler and calmer I became. I noticed that at the height of my panic attack, I'd go into the Yoga positions and stretch my muscles. The result was a sudden sense of calm. Don't take soy isoflavones in powder form where it is highly concentrated if you have breast cancer because it's not recommended. For those not at high risk of any condition, soy is supposed to be good for your arteries. I took soy products for chronic anxiety, and combined with yoga, here's how it stretched out my doubts.

Talk to professional nutritionists, health care professionals and compare their views with naturopaths and alternative nutrition counselors. Have a genetic test to see how your body reacts to various foods, vitamins, mineral build up. For example, does calcium raise your blood pressure or lower it?

Different people react in different ways. What ration of calcium to magnesium is best for you? That's why you need to talk to professionals trained in tailoring your foods and any other treatments to your individual genes.

Get tested for what is scientifically accurate about nutrition and genetic testing. Check out any companies with health care professionals. Find out what other patients/clients are saying about their own treatments. What works for you may not work for someone else. Stretching and walking in place worked wonders in the midst of a panic attack—at least for me.

Each time I did mild stretching with my legs and arms, anxiety would fade. A feeling of sending out waves of love to my worst enemy took over my body and mind. My dominant introverted feeling personality type emphasized values. I asked myself: Is this issue worth weakening my heart's pacemaker by an adrenaline bath? The answer was always, of course not.

Now, my body had to understand that feeling value at the molecular level as well. The best and healthiest answers came when I asked a value question, is it worth it?

Yoga, Tai Chi, and Qi Gong were the best event in my writing life and in stretching, balancing, and walking to relax. Stretching resulted in a feeling of calmness. Listening to calming music or chanting also felt relaxing during a panic episode.

The calming, meditative new age and ethnic music helped to relaxed me. Oddly, high-spirited belly dance music without too much drumming gave me a feeling of wellbeing, not panic. The drumming increased my heartbeat and raised my blood pressure. So I didn't choose music with a lot of fast drumming.

People's bodies react to the tempo of the music. If a music piece is only 60 beats a minute with a metronome, the human body responds to that beat and calms down to a feeling of relaxation. Your body eventually moves in sync with the music beats. That's why I choose slow music.

My whole body would physiologically react to the beat of the music. The slow beats, precisely music of 60 beats per minute brought me down to a relaxed normal feeling. Classical string and brass music of the 17th century felt the best along with new-age, stress-reduction, and relaxing music made for meditation. When calm, I liked bellydance or tribal dance music with a slow beat to stretch to. The focus of each movement emphasized keeping my balance. And when the rhythm changed, the bellydance hip-drop helped me focus on losing the stress.

◆　　◆　　◆

How to Make a More Nutritious Cookie—Vegan Cookie Recipe with Rice Bran, Oat, and Flax meal.

Low-sodium and only natural fruit sweetening … No bleached flour ingredients. Use oat bran, flax seed meal, and oatmeal instead of flour. No eggs, baking powder, soda, or dairy products.

The Recipe:

1 scoop rice protein powder (about 2 tablespoons)
1 tub tofu made with calcium sulfate instead of magnesium chloride (about a pound) or three egg whites, beaten until in stiff peaks like meringue
1/2 to 2/3 cup of pink grapefruit juice. Buy a freshly squeezed carton of juice or juice your own grapefruit.
1 cup walnuts
1/2 cup almonds
1/4 cup extra virgin olive oil cold pressed and not rancid or old.
1/2 cup frozen blueberries
1/2 cup frozen strawberries
1 cup oat bran
1 cup oat meal—old fashioned rolled oats uncooked
1/2-2/3 cup flax seed meal
1 tablespoon of lecithin granules (optional)

Place in a bowl the oat bran, protein powder, lecithin, and flax seed meal, stir, then finally the oat meal, then all the fruit and nut ingredients. In a blender blend the grapefruit juice and tofu. Pour into the large glass bowl.

Stir everything. Pour all ingredients into the bowl and mix with a large spoon. If you need more sweetness, consider fruit, but please go lightly here. You don't want sugar to raise those insulin levels. I like it without sweetener. Use pieces of fresh dates, chopped apples, or figs to sweeten more, if you require a sweeter taste.

You can serve with almond butter, peanut butter, or other high protein or nut butter topping if you wish. The addition of the Omega-3 oils in the form of flax seed meal, is helpful, and at least helped me. This is a nutritious nut and fruit cookie that can supplement a meal on the run.

Coat 2 or 3 cookie sheets with the extra virgin olive oil. (I use glass cookie sheets). Bake in a 350 degree F. oven for 40 minutes or from 30 to 45 minutes, until the undersides of the cookies are a light brown.

Use a metal spatula to lift the warm cookies and place into a cake dish or other glass bowl. Cover and let cool. The world's most nutritious cookie is served warm. It's delicious.

The key ingredient is the rice protein powder and the absence of granulated white sugar, fruit juice concentrate, or dairy fat.

◆   ◆   ◆

Raspberry/Carrot Vegan Cookie Recipe with Rice Bran, Oat, and Flax meal.

Low-sodium and only natural fruit sweetening. No bleached flour ingredients. Use oat bran, flax seed meal, and oat meal instead of flour. No eggs, baking powder, soda, or dairy products.

The Recipe:

2 scoops rice protein powder (about 2 tablespoons)
1 cup of unsweetened almond milk.
1/2 to 2/3 cup of frozen or fresh red raspberries blended with a cup of soy milk.
1 peeled banana
1 cup walnuts
1/2 cup almonds
1/4 cup extra virgin olive oil cold pressed and not rancid or old.
1/2 cup frozen blueberries
1/2 cup frozen strawberries
1/2 cup peeled baby carrots
1 cup oat bran
1 cup oat meal—old fashioned rolled oats uncooked
1/2-2/3 cup flax seed meal
1 tablespoon of lecithin granules

2 or 3 egg whites. Or if vegan substitute 1/2 tub tofu (blended to a creme) for eggs or 1/2 cup stewed prunes in their syrup and 2 tablespoons of lecithin granules if you don't eat egg whites.

In a blender blend the almond milk and fruit. Add the peeled baby carrots. Liquify. Taste it and it will taste like a rather tart soymilk product.

Pour into a large glass bowl. Add two or three egg whites to a bowl and add the soy milk and fruit blended to a thick smoothie consistency. Add to the bowl the oat bran, protein powder, lecithin, and flax seed meal, stir, then finally the oatmeal, then all the fruit and nut ingredients.

Mix in bowl. Or if you're a vegan, substitute 1/2 pound tub of tofu or 1/2 stewed prunes in their syrup and 2 tablespoons of lecithin granules for the egg whites that will hold the cookie paste together.

Stir everything. Pour all ingredients into the bowl and mix with a large spoon. If you need more sweetness, consider fruit, but please go lightly here. You don't want sugar to raise those insulin levels. I like it without sweetener.

You can serve with almond butter, peanut butter, or other high protein or nut butter topping if you wish. The addition of the Omega-3 oils in the form of flax seed meal, is helpful, and at least helped me. This is a nutritious nut and fruit cookie that can supplement a meal on the run.

Coat two or three cookie sheets with the olive oil. I use glass cookie sheets. Bake in a 350 degree F. oven for 40 minutes or from 30 to 45 minutes, until the undersides of the cookies are a light brown.

Use a metal spatula to lift the warm cookies and place into a cake dish or other glass bowl. Cover and let cool. The world's most nutritious cookie is served warm. It's delicious. The key ingredients are the rice bran and rice protein powder and the absence of granulated white sugar, fruit juice concentrate, or dairy fat.

◆   ◆   ◆

2

Too Scared To Leave Home, Speak in Public, or Answer the Phone

I dreamed that I danced on a lavish tropical cruise, a gift from my children. And there were four or more generations present in celebration of my zillionth wedding anniversary. Only I've never attended a wedding—never had an actual wedding of my own, and never wore a bridal gown. There's no way I could walk onto a ship without being hit with a bout of vertigo. Nor can I fly, drive, travel, or walk out of my home after sundown.

I'm too scared of people's hate and too scared of my body's fluctuations—that my body will betray me. And as far as my children giving me a gift of travel and fun, forget it. They call twice a year for five minutes. Not that I'd complain, mind you. I'm more concerned why some peoples' bodies betray them and what you as an individual can do about it, perhaps learn to thrive from analyzing the details of my experience.

Why do so many women betray other women they have never met in person and so many men back them up and believe them without thinking to write to the person being bullied by the largely female practice of exclusion? Too scared of people's hate to leave home or answer the phone, humor writer and Anna Magnani look-alike, I, yours truly, of Brooklyn's Bensonhurst and Borough Park, spent nearly thirty years with panic disorder, agoraphobia, and sociophobia—trapped in my home most, but not all of the time by a fear of people, heightened panic, and open spaces.

I have not left my home after sun down since 1987. It's too dangerous to wait at bus stops in the night. I can't afford taxis, and I'm too scared to ask a stranger for a ride. There are no relatives around that are able to drive. Based in my home, by choice again, after 5:00 PM, my work day in the creative arts begins online.

When the sun rises, my walking day begins outside wherever I can find the scent of a blooming tree.

Nondriver by choice, always I'd been afraid to fly, to travel, to go near water, afraid of the men walking the streets night, afraid to go far from home, afraid of the smell of fear. The panic washed over me as I watched the "angry poor" talking to themselves.

They'd pass me in the street and shout into my face, "Hey, old lady, got some change to spare for the homeless?" Then they'd spit out a cuss word and, bare-chested, whip their shirts, punching the air. I'd suppress body movements and walk on, stone-faced, but inside my body, the fear made my heart jump, and it wore me out too early.

The younger males would lash out at me merely for my looks, on public transportation. Why wasn't it all right to be a woman alone outside walking from the bus to home and have a scar on my face all my youth that now folded neatly into my age-wise wrinkles?

For nearly thirty years, on and off, I remained trapped at home with agoraphobia and panic disorder. Walking in place finally cut me free to walk again, at least in the daylight hours, outside my home. By doing the motion inside that I could not do outside, the pathways in my brain imprinted so to speak with the notion that walking is familiar. Then I increased the walking to Tai Chi exercises, then Qi Gong to stimulate the immune system by exercising the "cleaning action" of the lymph nodes.

Finally, I began to apply the stretching that calmed me during a panic attack (stretching one foot) to gentle Yoga stretching. These simpler forms of Yoga and meditation designed for older individuals kept improving my ability to walk outside the home and not feel so scared. Later, I added slow bellydancing and tribal dancing to healing music and continued the Tai Chi for balance.

How the Panic Began in 1963

The panic that eventually kept me trapped in my home for years actually began after being brutally strangled in the snow near my home by a man who followed me home at night from the subway (tube). The sound of a creaking window saved me at the last moment only because a senior citizen wanted fresh air, and the sudden noise frightened him away. This event happened in a New York City Subway when I was age 21.

Then at age 22, I took a train back from a vacation in Asbury Park, New Jersey returning to New York. I was married at the time and two-months pregnant. It was 1964, and the movie, *Cleopatra* was all over town. I had tinted my auburn hair black; made my green eyes up to look Egyptian, and thought I looked like Liz Taylor when I gazed back at myself in the mirror. In August of 1964 I was married, two months pregnant, and then my self-image melted.

A man, who I call the neo-Nazi, told me not to cross between cars while the train was in motion until the train stopped in Elizabeth, New Jersey. He wasn't the conductor. He was a passenger with his wife. I couldn't understand why he would order me to "wait 'till the train stopped in Elizabeth." I told him I was pregnant and returning from the john, and needed to get back to my seat or my husband, an Omar Sharif look-alike, and mother, a Joan Collins look-alike, riding in the next car would think I became ill in the bathroom. He ignored me.

So I passed in front of him to return to my seat. I didn't brush him or touch his luggage or anything. There was no conductor around, and normally the right procedure is when you walk from one train car to the next to use the bathroom, it's regular procedure to walk back to your seat in the next car by opening and closing the easily sliding doors.

There were no train rules broken, of course. Because I didn't defer and defied his command, by walking past him to reach the next car and return silently to my seat and husband, he grabbed my head in a vise-like grip with his hand and knee, squeezed, trying to crush my head between his knee and the wall of the train causing me great pain in the skull, and beat the hell out of me by squeezing my head.

The pain of my head being squeezed first between his large hands and then between his knees was unbearable. Then he held me so I couldn't move and kicked me hard at the base of the spine while he yelled, "you dirty Jew." I went flying forward into the next car while his wife eyed my wedding ring as I faced her for a moment, and quietly smirked, "let her go, dear."

The man's wife or female companion had the sweetest controlled voice as she looked up at me behind the fishnet veil of her pillbox hat. The two reminded me of the painting, "Gothic American."

He sported top-headed baldness with black hair around the rim of his ears, staring black eyes, and pale, ecru skin. She looked the same with curled brown hair and wrinkles above her thin lips. The words, "dirty Jew," rang in my head. I walked back to my seat two cars down and never said a word to my husband or mother.

My then husband would have returned and started a fight. My mother had just gotten out of the hospital and was recuperating. For the next twenty years I never said a word ... to anyone. My fear of being Jewish went inward and increased. When I wrote about my experience, some women accused me of being "a man-hater."

The next day I stopped trying to look like Elizabeth Taylor in *Cleopatra*. I bleached the black tint out of my brown hair and made it bright red. With the freckles and hazel green eyes, I announced to the mirror that I now looked Welsh. Funny, how nobody noticed my convex nose, I surmised, when my hair was medium ash blonde or Killarney russet.

A few times during my teenage years in Brooklyn, some Puerto Ricans asked me whether I were Scottish or Irish. One black man tried to strangle me without asking what I was first. He only asked where my money was. A white man asked me once where the synagogue was, but I remember seeing him on TV as one of the skinheads taken into custody.

He was teasing me. First he asked me whether I needed help crossing the street and called me old lady. When I told him my age as if to say, I'm not that old, he brought up the Jewish lady part, emphatically with fury and frustration.

By then, so many years ago, I welcomed age 60, turned around, and told him this face is what Mediterranean people look like. At that point in a public street in a Mexican area of San Diego, I felt disgusted and so tired of people asking me where I'm from and what I am.

Almost every time I opened my mouth I was asked when I had come from New York. In one city, I walked into a seminar in women's history and heard that the professor had received death threats when he was appointed chairman of the Jewish Studies department that sponsored the free seminars at a university open to the public.

Most people who showed up were over age sixty and a few history students. So much for freedom of speech in a state university hall, it seems. The next lecture I went to was on quilting. The teacher never got any threats teaching crafts. All I went there for was to make a friend and find some place to belong. I still don't belong anywhere and have not yet made an attempt to make friends, although I want to. It became harder to find friends after age sixty-three, and I never learned to drive—too scared to take tests anymore.

It's nearly fifty years since I left Brooklyn. Why is it so important? I have been housebound on and off all these 30+ years. I have never learned to drive a car. I'm afraid to fly or travel very far from home. I don't answer the phone. I'm afraid when the phone rings that someone is going to say something hurtful or ask for donations or put my name on a list to automatically receive something I don't want to buy because I've almost outlived my money.

The only people that ever call anyway ask me to vote for someone, to donate, or to buy something I really don't need. In my childhood the phone only rang when somebody called to announce the day and time of an old relative's funeral or to sell something we could never afford to buy. I'm so scared I jump when the phone rings.

It usually is bad news, or a scam trying to trap me because they think I'm too old to enjoy anything they have judged that I'd outlived. What's it like to be more or less housebound with the housewife's 'gene' (that even men can inherit) for more than 30 years and find solace in writing and watching travel videos?

Why do so many women betray other women and work, and so many poor men and middle-aged women call still stranger older women upon first meeting them, "mama or granny?" The litmus test of humanity is how we treat others that are not empowered to promote or enrich us with material goods, but can offer spiritual inspiration to be all that we can be and to do the best with what we have.

◆   ◆   ◆

During those years trapped at home with agoraphobia, chronic anxiety, and panic disorder, I kept thinking, "What's my core identity?" Each morning I rose to fear. I asked myself then "What does it feel like to live disguised as an Arab housewife for seven years in a Jewish neighborhood in Brooklyn?" Here I sat: the great grand daughter of a lineage of scholarly rabbis reared by secular parents that broke away totally from organized religion. My mother and I would attend Christian churches.

I had been taken to see what all religions practiced on each of their holy days, and I had to choose for myself. My secular parents made it clear that any books written about organized religion or secularism were all written by men.

So I focused on the one book written by a woman, *Mary Baker Eddy's Science and Health with Key to the Scriptures*. That book became my religion. And I made it as secular as I could by focusing on "divine intelligence" for any mention of deities. Perhaps her book would help me stretch, dance, and walk my way out of agoraphobia and panic disorder that had kept me trapped at home for nearly 30 years.

I still can't drive, fly, or go in a boat due to my inner ear problems with vertigo (the result of an auto accident in which I sat in the back seat while my late first husband drove the car). One smash in the head in a car accident, and again I became trapped at home by on-and-off vertigo that lasts a few days when an episode hits, usually when I'm under stress.

Genes are destiny, I had been told, but you can switch bad genes off and turn good genes on with certain foods, nutrients, exercises, and attitudes. That's where Eddy's outlook helped to relieve the stress of living in an environment of chronic anxiety. My short 5-HTT gene set me up to easily experience anxiety. Reading all I could about how genes work to determine what you do with your life helped me understand that environment works also, but in a more limited way.

The fact that my parents never had finished elementary school didn't stop me from eventually receiving a graduate degree. I worked full time, earned the tuition money myself, and went to university classes between six and ten o'clock in the evenings.

Anxiety increased dramatically each time I got mugged, harassed, or assaulted on the subway commuting from work or college. That was New York City in 1959-1964.

Interestingly, agoraphobia and panic disorder hit full blast when I had my first child, and my late first husband began the wife-beating that started the day before I had to go to the hospital to have my first child. Post-traumatic stress syndrome hit me from three angles—my father's continuing elder rage at my mother, assaults from strangers on the subway, and my husband's beatings and threats. To analyze how my genetic predisposition to anxiety influenced my life at home, my mother's early life became the first place to start.

Mom had come from a broken home in which she had been given away at the age of two when her parents divorced. She had been beaten so many times in the 1910 era by people of a wide variety of backgrounds that the stories she told me as a young child were filled with fear about one's core identity.

Maintaining a low profile became most important. The outlook repeated daily emphasized how I could be 'saved' by meeting a "good provider." Mom's words which she attributed to hearing her own mother say to her step-dad when mom met her biological mother for the first time at the age of 19 went like this: "A 'lady' is a woman attractive enough to find a rich man who is kind and slow to anger. He will be a good provider. She will feel safe in his presence. When he drives, he will not cuss out other drivers out loud with his wife sitting next to him in fear.

A 'woman' is unable to find a good provider or a man who is slow to anger. She will work and pay the bills, and he will put her down to pick himself up. He will intimidate her, keep her off balance, and make her cry each time they go for a ride, especially if she complains that he cusses loudly when he drives and another driver does something he doesn't like." (That's the difference between a woman and a lady.)

It's true, I surmised, because both my husbands treated me like a 'woman' and not like a 'lady.' And grandma's second husband treated her just like my husbands treated me.

Mom told me that when she visited her own mother when age 19, her step dad would yell, "No, you're a woman," each time grandma would shout back, "No, I'm a lady." That's how genes interplay with environment to create generations of women whose words are so similar in angry marriages.

Have the 'anxiety' gene, so to speak, plays a role in not growing, moving on, or looking for what the Bible describes the Creator as being 'slow to anger.' But men are slow to anger only if they have inherited the 'calm' gene, or more succinctly, the calming branch of their nervous system working with a long, not a short version of their 5-HTT gene that causes hyperactivity in the brain's fear center.

When the entire family has this 'short' gene, including husband and wife, well, you have a picture, regardless of the changing environment. How much could the environment change to override the genetic predisposition?

You'd have to marry the perfect, loving husband. Where are you going to meet such a man when your own family is steeped in poverty and you father also has deep anxiety issues as a World War I disabled veteran? In New York, men that are good providers and slow to anger look to marry into similar families.

Even a matchmaker would be afraid to place a gentleman from the type of family I would have wanted into my poverty-stricken, anxiety-saturated secular family. I always thought my university graduate degree would be a passport to the middle class. But the door to the middle class remained closed.

The only way it could open would be if I married into it. But I never did find that "good provider." As for a job, when I started looking, the Baby Boom generation had already filled all the good teaching jobs. The few years I spent at home raising my two children to age four and five had used up the head start or lead time I had on the Boomers' race to employment. And by the time I started looking to earn income, agoraphobia had trapped me solidly at home for many years to come.

A woman goes to college, but will her genes predispose her to postpartum agoraphobia and panic disorder? If she has a degree, what good is it if she's trapped at home for years by anxiety and a defective autonomic nervous system where the slightest work stress causes her to panic and shake with fear?

The words created visual imagery that I remembered into old age. What I heard in middle childhood emphasized that the only man who'd marry a woman as "ugly, scarred, and large, convex-nosed" as me (to use a relative's words) would be only if "I became a wealthy professional or ran a large business and had cash." But since I had statistically, only a one to three percent "chance of becoming rich enough to enter the upper middle class," the person who married me, most likely would be a schlemiel, defined as an insecure man with low self-esteem and less education, common sense, or intelligence than his wife.

One day some angry, low-self esteemed, future wife-beating schlemiel out there will marry me, pay the bills, and hug me every morning for the first three months of marriage. A schlemazel is the guy who spills his soda pop from a theater balcony onto the head of the schlemiel below, the receiver, usually a giver at the beginning of a courtship. The schlemazel, a taker all during the courtship, marries a rich man or woman with low self esteem. The schlemiel, generous, insecure, and also with low self esteem, marries a poor man or woman, of course, also with low self esteem. *She can't take care of herself, and he can't take care of her.*

The bullied schlemiel, like the bullying schlemazel, is absorbed in his own looks, hurt, and anger. Only the schlemiel bullies women with low self esteem, low confidence, and the fear of future low income. The schlemazel bullies men and women because he remembers the angry world of his childhood.

Isn't a good provider what every mother wants and passes on to her daughters—especially when paid jobs and other income are scarce and the woman is physically unable to leap tall buildings when roundly pregnant?

What does it feel like to live disguised as an Arab housewife for seven years in a Jewish neighborhood in Brooklyn followed by decades trapped on-and-off at home with agoraphobia long after being divorced when it is supposed to be all right again to be what makes the world a kinder and gentler place, what heals and repairs?

It feels like by doing something differently, I could inspire someone to change the world in a positive way for all sides. I wish I had a close, loving, warm, joy-filled family. Don't we all? It takes work, but it can be done. Only the Arab divorced me and took the children, as is the custom in his culture, but not in mine. That was forty years ago.

Maybe now that's why I like to watch big, loud Greek weddings, Italian weddings, Lebanese weddings, Jewish weddings, and Armenian weddings. The music sounds like joy. It's so far from the experience of being the daughter of a battered wife who turns on the TV to see movies about women preyed upon by men or beasts that hurt because they have been hurt. I turned on the TV for role model therapy.

That's why my favorite movie was *"My Big, Fat Greek Wedding."* I look towards the characters in that movie as role models for how families with a core identity could interact with joy of life. I long for a close, warm, loving family, a big family that dances and plays ethnic music and serves tasty food. Invite me to your ethnic wedding, and I shall bring you a gift and eat well.

If you want a joy-of-life family, you can become a world changer. It's someone who influences people close by or far away in space or time to do something they would not have done or to do it differently than they would have done it. World changers influence people positively or negatively.

Mom once said, "Don't try to change the world. It's all genetic." I wonder whether genes determine each person's fortune unequally in the financial arena as in the "survival of the fittest theory?" Science might change genes with gene therapy, but can everyone experience joy of life equally, or is joy also inherited? I'm banking on joy.

Paternal Great Grandma

"Belle W___, born in 1861, from Lodz, Poland, maybe lived in Brest-Litovsk, *perhap*s a distant relative of C___ W____, President of Israel," the genealogist revealed with pride to my aunt. Belle W_____ is my mother's dad's mother's maiden name. Belle married I____ T_____, whose son, born in 1881, C____ M____ T_____, had Anglicized his name to H____ T_____.

My mom after fifty, looked more Irish than, but the spitting image of a female version of Jackie Gleason. Mom at age 21 on a photo looked like Joan Collins, and at 35, more like Loretta Young. Mom had been so afraid of being rejected or beaten by telling non-Jews she was Jewish, that she'd led two lives in our home. Our spiritual life felt so Christian and/or agnostic at times with me, but Jewish with my brother and dad.

Mom and I happily spent our afternoons a few times a year going to a variety of Christian churches—the Dutch reformed, Christian Science Reading Rooms, Episcopal, Greek Orthodox, Italian Catholic, Quaker, Methodist, Unitarian, Congregationalist, Ethical Culture, Religious Science, Science of Mind, Baptist, Evangelical, Spiritualist, Humanist, Tibetan Buddhist, and you name it as long as it included 1950-style new age meditation, Yoga, and painting of mandalas.

We loved to float between churches, especially to look at and savor the decorations on Christmas and Easter. I loved going to Mass at Saint Patrick's Cathedral in New York on Christmas. Then I'd come home and walk through the Hasidic neighborhoods in Brooklyn's Borough Park and imagine what it would be like to be part of a big family that eats and prays together instead of watching dad punch mom in the chest.

Sometimes I wandered off to the Sephardic synagogues or the Hasidic neighborhoods. With the Hasidim, I felt in the presence of real family where men didn't beat their wives. Later I found out domestic violence cuts through all ethnic, economic, and religious groups. It's a toss up between domestic violence instead of peace in the home and the housing laws as to why I enjoyed going to so many churches.

Ultimately, I sought a healing experience. The goal centered upon finding a church to understand the philosophy that turns on the gene for spontaneous healing based on a faith that assures us we are loved, wanted, cherished and here for a good purpose such as healing and repairing the world in some individualized way.

I wanted to be told that the parallel universes of chaos had some order for a reason—such as to care for one another. In practical terms, my desire to practice two or more religions at once focused on the housing laws which in the 1950s focused on what ethnic and religious group you espoused. By choosing an easy-to-remember name and attending a Protestant church, by tinting my brown hair blonde, the notion that someday when I grow up that I might own a house in California became closer to reality.

I wanted to fit into the majority group, to assimilate but still keep my vegetarian choices, to marry without restrictions, and to reason that if the Creator created this universe and all of its intelligent beings, it's only logical that each would be created equal in his or her ability to buy a house anywhere in the country of one's citizenship. I 'believe' in evolution and genomics.

We once were chimps and intermarried with chimps even when we branched off to the line that eventually led to becoming human. That's why we have genes so close to chimps today. Like chimps, some go on the warpath. We are in the midst of evolving—still too close to the cave, and not yet able to control space, time, and starlight. But we will someday be able to bend those light and gravity waves. My thoughts on life purpose are related to the 1940s housing laws.

The housing laws years ago didn't allow Jews, Armenians, Middle Easterners, Eastern Europeans and nonwhites to buy housing in certain parts of the country that my family coveted, particularly in some of the palm latitudes such as La Jolla, California.

Housing laws changed after 1950, but my core identity either had to change or didn't change with the new housing laws. I don't understand housing laws. I'm an American. That's my identity.

I don't see why I have to bleach my hair and change my name to practice being an American and buy a house anywhere in America. I'm a secular American who respects all peoples. So what did changing my name, bleaching my hair, and fitting in have to do with me coming down with postpartum agoraphobia that trapped me in my home at various times for nearly three decades? It's all about hormone fluctuations, a short 5-HTT gene, and fearing people wouldn't like me going to a different church each week to savor the delicious sermons that made me feel as if I had a loving family, of course putting a donation in the plate each time. I enjoy all of humanity, but why couldn't my family buy a house in La Jolla during the 1940s?

By the time I moved from Brooklyn to La Jolla in 1967, nobody cared what church I went to, how much I spent legally changing my name, or what hue of highlights I bleached into my chestnut tresses. By then I became housebound with agoraphobia, and with all the efforts I made to lessen my Brooklyn accent, 'looking' southern Italian happened to be fine. After all, Italy is not in Eastern Europe.

How do you look southern Italian? You look like portraits of aristocratic ancient Romans—wavy brown hair, convex nose, hazel eyes, fair to medium complexion. And you wear hair nets spun of fine gold thread. Besides, I have enough relatives that married Romans and Greeks in modern times. So we all fit into the great salad bowl of America, and nobody gives a care. It's not important. What counts is how we treat one another. Imagine what would have happened to my dream if we really did try to move to California in the 1940s, my early elementary school years.

According to the article, "Flaw in the Jewel: Housing Discrimination Against Jews in La Jolla, CA,"—American Jewish History 84:3 (1996) 189-219, when Dr. Jonas Salk, the first Jew to move to La Jolla, CA moved next door to a non-Jew, that person put his/her house on the market.

What's my core identity? What do I have to be to buy a house in the Garden of Eden—beachside, California? So we all turned Protestant and tinted chestnut hair medium ash blonde.

The family's green eyes fitted in perfectly with our new English names. Why did we have to do this to buy a house? Even my matrilineal mtDNA—my ancient female ancestor several thousand years old says I'm not 'Jewish'—but Scandinavian or North Central European. My mtDNA is most common in Norway, Scotland, and Finland. So who am I? I'm part of the human race, and that should be all that's required.

My great, great grandfather was a scholarly rabbi. I should by all rights be part of the pedigreed Hasidim. Or should I? I'm the only Jewish member of my family left, and I've always worshipped alone. In the past fifty years, not one relative has contacted me asking to be my pen pal and/or best friend.

Why? I am poor, over age 65, and have married more than three decades ago a Protestant agnostic and Spiritualist whose relatives came from England to America in 1632. So what? Why is it important if the Creator created and loves everyone equally. I believe the intelligence that created everything is love, is consciousness, and is intelligence. It is not filled with human emotions of anger, but is pure love of life as expanding eternally throughout the various universes.

What I miss most is belonging to a family, but there's no one left. So I have to embrace all the religions the surviving younger generation has embraced. No one gets left out, but no one has included me. I'm pushing 70, and I don't have a family who ever visits.

My paternal great grandmother born around 1834 in Bialystok, Poland, her daughter, Anna Kutkowski, "The Cat"—born around 1854, my dad, one of nine children born (last in birth order) in 1894, my mom, from another land, born in 1904, whom dad married in 1926, and I born before World War Two, all were and are tired of being beaten up for looking Jewish. We've had it.

We're not tailoring our noses or tinting our hair any more. We look Middle Eastern, and we are tired of Middle Eastern people, whatever their religion getting beaten up for looking like they just stepped out of Babylon or Beirut.

My mother looked like the actress, Joan Collins in the movie "The Egyptian."

I look like the sultry Italian actress, Anna Magnani. We are all Mediterranean-type women descended from Neolithic farmers of the grain belt born from women who lived centuries in Bialystok, Poland, and we are tired of getting our ears boxed for not always looking like Swedish milk maids in spite of some of us born with red hair, light eyes, fair complexions, and freckles.

No matter how red or blonde our hair is or how green, blue, or hazel our eyes and light our skin, one look at our paternal side's large family's convex noses, and the shouts go up half in Yiddish, "Favus, Favus, she gotta longa nuz." So who started the *war* of exclusion against attractive women with convex curves—noses or bellies? Is asymmetry visionary?

Convexity is age. Concavity is infancy. Babies have concave curves. Old people may have convex curves. So many parts grow more convex with age, but start out concave at birth. Does convexity release hormones that stimulate the fear of aging and mortality?

With my metabolic syndrome, a convex nose and a convex belly spelled the need not to fix it with plastic surgery, because that would not say convex is beautiful. It's better for the world to say convex is okay. You don't have to be concave to be pretty, loved, rich, or happy. It's fine to be yourself. Convex is not a deformity. It happens when a round head marries a long head, and the child becomes convex in face. And that's part of the normal tapestry of diversity.

Would you tell a person of another race to have plastic surgery to fit the ideal of beauty in your own race? No. All over the world symmetry is beautiful, regardless of race, if there is such a thing, which there is not. We're part of the human race.

Why should it take agoraphobia—the fear of meeting people, of going outside to teach me that it is okay to look what my ethnic ancestry is all about without a total stranger approaching me to smash me in the face or even tell me what I already know about my appearance, age, or economic status?

And who enriched my tapestry? How many tribes are in my temporary container? Why is concave crucial and convex curved? My journey was in search of a core identity, but it led to something transcending even that—a link with all peoples through universal archetypes. What made us what we are besides the changing climate?

The earliest tales my mother wove, starting about the age of three, was about when the German mothers boxed her ears. It wasn't in Europe, but in Albany, New York. My mother was born in an old house in Albany, New York in 1904 to a woman from Bessarabia, Romania, (Ashkenazic Jews and Germans migrated from Poland, Ukraine, Latvia, Belarus, Germany, and Lithuania to Bessarabia in the 18th century), and a blond, silver-eyed man who looked almost exactly like Clark Gable, from Lodz, Poland. Dad's parents came from Bialystok, Poland in the late 19th century. If I'm supposed to be so pink-and-white Polish, how come I look like I just stepped out of Beirut?

How I am mixed, only my mtDNA and nuclear DNA says, and my maternal DNA says I'm Northern European. It's not important how I'm mixed, only that I'm not mixed up. Isn't everyone mixed? Even Arabs have mixtures of DNA from Europeans from people escaping the ravages of the last ice age to the Northern European crusaders who married Lebanese women in medieval times?

And what a hoax Hitler made about Nordic looks when he hired the grand Mufti of Jerusalem to lead his Bosnian officers in Europe. Certainly the grand Mufti of Jerusalem looked as Lebanese if one can look Lebanese as I do. So it makes no difference where you come from. If you have one round-headed parent and one long-headed parent, the child will look the stereotypical caricature of Hittite, Semite, and Aramaic, Armenian, Kurd, Adriatic, Roman, West coast Greek, or Persian. So why are ethnic looks so important to you that you'd create a housing code in certain California cities forbidding anyone with convex curves to buy a house in that spot from the 1950s counting backwards? Oh, it's East Europeans that were included in the housing codes? What about my relatives from Finland and Eastern Sweden—the Baltic sisters? Hmm?

When my mother was two years old, her parents divorced and her mother gave her away to her father. He took her to Philadelphia. There, she was raised by a redheaded stepmother from Vienna, Austria and Odessa, Russia. As I grew up, my mother would tell me story after story of how she was beaten by hate crimes in the U.S. as a child. African-Americans beat her for having pink skin and silver eyes.

Whites beat her for "looking Jewish" and having black and curly hair along with Mongolian features, supposedly inherited from the Khazars and the peoples of the Silk Road. And, gee, nobody beat her for looking like my mother. When she was ten in the fifth grade, she asked a fellow student, "Do I look Jewish?"

The student replied, "You got the map of Jerusalem printed on your face."

On and on, mom would talk to me, and each time, there was another tale of how she played with neighbor kids and their German mothers would box her ears and call her epithets with the word "Jew" in them. The stereotype is of anyone from a Mediterranean country or the Caucasus Mountains who happens to have the profile of King Sargon of Babylon as his mask portrayed thousands of years ago, or a Sicilian profile with fair skin, light eyes, and dark hair. So why is it important?

What's not symmetrical enough for you? Well neither was the profile of King Tut, or Pharaoh Ramses, (may his mummy rest in peace) and nobody puts his finger to his nose and curls it convexly, except in a 1971 "All in the Family" episode followed by familiar canned laughter.

My early childhood experienced World War II, in Brooklyn. We lived in a four-family house near Kings Highway. Between the ages of three and five, not only did mom tell me about the holocaust in Europe, because I was born in 1941, but she would rock me in her arms when I was three, sweating in anxiety, as she sang to me about the bombs that were coming to fall on New York pretty soon.

There were lights out air raid drills, and always she told me the bombs were coming to fall, and they never did. The sweating, the anxiety was there anyway, almost as if they had come. Then she'd tell me about how the Irish and German Americans used to beat her for looking Jewish in the neighborhoods. She grew up (aged 10 to 14) during World War One. The street we lived on had been mostly Jewish on one side and partly southern Italian on the other, and almost never the twain met or spoke to one another.

Mom was a battered wife. Not only did I experience the holocaust from her stories, but the battles inside my home. My father, age 47 when I was born, and my brother, 13 years older than I, beat mom. There were terrible fights. I hid in my room and drew cartoons of them fighting.

One day my father smashed my piano and violin and all my birthday toys because I kicked him out of the bed I slept in with my mother when he tried to enter the bed in the middle of the night to have sex with my mother.

I was nine, and I told him to get out. He slept in the room next door in twin beds with my older brother in the room. The rule stood firm: men with men, women with women—throughout my parent's marriage. And dad beat mom.

She told me about how he beat her when she came home from the hospital with me a week old, and he punched her in the chest, and I fell from her arms into the snow. She had told him to hurry up and take the baby's picture because I was turning blue from the cold wind and snow.

My father always smashed things with hammers and axes. I was afraid someday he'd get me and kill me. Mom told me how much she worried, about everything, and most of all how awful it was to be Jewish and be beaten for looking Jewish. As I grew up, I began to look in the mirror and wonder whether I looked Jewish. I had a "Caspian Sea Nose."

My cousins told me "I looked very Semitic." So I began to make myself up to look like an ancient Egyptian, eye makeup, black wig or hair tint, and costume.

As I grew into a teenager, I took up the Turkish Belly dance, the Egyptian cane dance, the Moroccan dance, and the Zamba-Mora, a mixture of Flamenco and Moorish. My ballet lessons started at the age of five. By the age of eleven I danced on point—(toe).

At nine I gave a performance in ballet, a solo on the stage at my elementary school. At seven I started violin lessons and at nine, piano lessons. Music became my life. At thirteen I added voice lessons. I went on to graduate from college as a creative writing major, fine art minor, with second minors in psychology and anthropology. I was into ethnomusicology and linguistics. My hobby was astronomy and illustration ... writing poetry, novels.

Then, at 22, I took a train back from a vacation in Asbury Park, returning to New York. I was married at the time, to a non-Jew. It was 1964, and the movie, *Cleopatra* was all over town. I had tinted my hair black; made my eyes up to look Egyptian, and thought I looked like Liz Taylor when I gazed back at myself in the mirror. In August of 1964 I was married, two months pregnant, and then my self image melted.

A man, who I call the neo-Nazi, told me not to cross between cars while the train was in motion until the train stopped in Elizabeth, New Jersey. He wasn't the conductor. He was a passenger with his wife. I couldn't understand why he would order me to "wait 'till the train stopped in Elizabeth." I told him I was pregnant and returning from the john, and needed to get back to my seat or my husband and mother riding in the next car would think I became ill in the bathroom.

He ignored me. So I passed in front of him to return to my seat. I didn't brush him or touch his luggage or anything. There was no conductor around, and normally the right procedure is when you walk from one train car to the next to use the bathroom, it's regular procedure to walk back to your seat in the next car by opening and closing the easily sliding doors.

There were no train rules broken, of course. Because I didn't defer and defied his command, by walking past him to reach the next car and return silently to my seat and husband, he grabbed my head in a vise-like grip with his hand and knee, squeezed, trying to crush my head between his knee and the wall of the train causing me great pain in the skull, and beat the hell out of me by squeezing my head.

The pain of my head being squeezed first between his large hands and then between his knees was unbearable. Then he held me so I couldn't move and kicked me hard at the base of the spine while he yelled, "you dirty Jew." I went flying forward into the next car while his wife eyed my wedding ring as I faced her for a moment, and quietly smirked, "let her go, dear."

She had the sweetest controlled voice as she looked up at me behind the fish-net veil of her pillbox hat. The two reminded me of the painting, "Gothic American." He was bald, black hair around the rim of his ears, staring black eyes, pale skin. She looked the same with curled brown hair and wrinkles above her thin lips. The words, "dirty Jew," rang in my head. I walked back to my seat two cars down and never said a word to my husband or mother.

My husband would have returned and started a fight. My mother had just gotten out of the hospital and was recuperating. For the next twenty years I never said a word … to anyone. My fear of being Jewish went inward and increased. When I wrote about my experience, some women accused me of being "a man-hater."

The next day I stopped trying to look like Elizabeth Taylor in *Cleopatra*. I bleached the black tint out of my brown hair and made it bright red. With the freckles and hazel green eyes, I announced to the mirror that I now looked Welsh. Funny, how nobody noticed my convex nose, I surmised, when my hair was medium ash blonde or Killarney russet.

A few times during my teenage years in Brooklyn, some Puerto Ricans asked me whether I were Scottish or Irish. One black man tried to strangle me without asking what I was first. He only asked where my money was. A white man asked me once where the synagogue was, but I remember seeing him on TV as one of the skinheads taken into custody.

He was teasing me. First he asked me whether I needed help crossing the street and called me old lady. When I told him my age as if to say, I'm not that old, he brought up the Jewish lady part, emphatically with fury and frustration.

I was over age 60-something then and turned around and told him this face is what Mediterranean people look like. At that point in a public street in a Mexican area of San Diego, I was disgusted and just tired of people asking me where I'm from and what I am. Every time I opened my mouth I was asked when I had come from New York. In one city, I walked into a seminar in Jewish history and heard that the professor had received death threats when he was appointed chairman of the Jewish Studies department that sponsored the free seminars at a university open to the public.

Most people who showed up were over age sixty and a few history students. So much for freedom of speech in a state university hall, it seems. The next lecture I went to was on quilting. The teacher never got any threats teaching crafts. All I went there for was to make a friend and find some place to belong. I still don't belong anywhere and have not yet made an attempt to make friends, although I want to. It became harder to find friends after age sixty-three, and I never learned to drive—too scared to take tests anymore.

It's more than forty years since I left Brooklyn. Why is it so important? I seldom speak in public, but talk to my video camera frequently. Then I let the videos become available to individuals seeking information.

I've become a recluse to have some semblance of serenity. Better to be alone than to be 'pecked.' On the Internet people stop asking about my New York accent online.

What is Jewish supposed to look like, an Assyrian king of 3,500 years ago?

Why do most Assyrian Christians look so much like me? With what group does my nuclear DNA or (matrilineal) mtDNA cluster?

Why can't we all accept one another's diversity without asking, without making it so important to know what someone's core identity is in privacy. I'm not your egg donor, so why ask? Nearly each time I open my mouth someone asks me when I left New York. I've been out of New York since 1965.

The man on the train who beat me didn't ask my name or look to see whether I wore a cross or a star or anything else. For a moment I wanted to say, "I'm Maltese. This is the face of Malta, or Naples, or Istanbul, or Crete." Perhaps my 38 college units in anthropology would have come in handy at that moment. But I said nothing for decades after that event.

So scared was my mother of being Jewish that she first joined the Dutch reformed (Protestant) church in Brooklyn and took me there when I was nine. We landed in the Christian Science church for decades. I also went to many other churches in the neighborhood. I liked the Science of Mind, the Religious Science, the Spiritualist, and the new age churches.

I liked the Episcopal Church because I could meditate in the quietness and be at one with the universe. At the Catholic Church, the nun once said to me, "I don't think you're Catholic. You look Jewish. What's your name?" I replied, "Angelica," because we lived near an Italian neighborhood, and I used to ask my Christian friends to donate their old rosaries to me because I collected them for those who needed them.

I loved holding the rosaries because they gave me peace. I realized all religions stream from one religion—the realization that life is part of a great brilliance, an intelligence with a goal—that life will persist in all the parallel universes. And that the goal is the growing toward consciousness and understanding of how to work with nature, time, and space.

I saw religion as links on a chain knowing we all come from and go to the same place. A loving God would not have created people in the first place unless he, she, or it, the Creator or designer sent us to the original source of life equally and took us from that original source of life to be born again and again.

I wondered how many different people wrote the Bible over so many years with all those Bible codes, predictions, inconsistencies, and contradictions, but thought it was great to have all that control over people who really would do you wrong. The Almighty's greatest gift to us is the freedom to choose for all the people seeking the highest right for the good of everyone in every universe where life exists.

◆   ◆   ◆

3

Post Traumatic Stress

I still think of myself as a descendant of people who lived in ancient Greece and the old Greek islands and colonies. My paternal great grandmother born around 1834 in Bialystok, Poland, her daughter, Anna Katkowski, "The Cat"—born around 1854, my dad, one of nine children born (last in birth order) in 1894, my mom, from another land, born in 1904, whom dad married in 1926, and I born before World War Two, all were and are tired of being beaten up for looking Jewish. We've had it.

We're not tailoring our noses or tinting our hair any more. We look Middle Eastern, and we are tired of Middle Eastern people, whatever their religion getting beaten up for looking like they just stepped out of Babylon or Beirut.

My mother looked like the actress, Joan Collins in the movie "The Egyptian." I look like the sultry Italian actress, Anna Magnani. We are all Mediterranean-type women descended from Neolithic farmers of the grain belt born from women who lived centuries in Bialystock, Poland, and we are tired of getting our ears boxed for not always looking like Swedish milk maids in spite of some of us born with red hair, light eyes, fair complexions, and freckles. No matter how red our hair is or how green, blue, or hazel our eyes and light our skin, one look at our large, convex noses, and the shouts go up half in Yiddish, "Favus, Favus, she gotta longa nuz."

So who enriched my tapestry? How many tribes are in my temporary container? At the cellular level I have a cultural and biological component. Why did those two components lead me to spend seven years in an Arab Jewish intermarriage to see how the other side lives? Why did I spend seven years disguised as an Arab housewife in a Brooklyn Jewish neighborhood and then in California? And why did I finally marry an Anglo-Saxon?

My journey was in search of a core identity, but it led to something transcending even that—a link with all peoples through universal archetypes. What made us what we are besides the changing climate?

The earliest tales my mother wove, starting about the age of three, was about when the German mothers boxed her ears. It wasn't in Europe, but in Albany, New York. My mother was born in an old house in Albany, New York in 1904 to a woman from Bessarabia, Romania, (Ashkenazic Jews and Germans migrated from Poland, Ukraine, Latvia, Belarus, Germany, and Lithuania to Bessarabia in the 18th century), and a blond, silver-eyed man who looked almost exactly like Clark Gable, from Lodz, Poland. Dad's parents came from Bialystock, Poland in the late 19th century. If I'm supposed to be so pink-and-white Polish, how come I look like I just stepped out of Beirut?

I'm probably mixed. How mixed, only my DNA says, and my maternal DNA says I'm Northern European. So where's my core identity? Do I look on the paternal side and try to guess how many genes I share with Arabs compared to Northern Europeans? Is it important? No, it is not as much as in finding my core identity. I'm looking instead for the cultural components of my DNA rather than solely the biological components. I am what music heals me.

When my mother was two years old, her parents divorced and her mother gave her away to her father. He took her to Philadelphia. There, she was raised by a redheaded stepmother from Vienna, Austria and Odessa, Russia. As I grew up, my mother would tell me story after story of how she was beaten by hate crimes in the U.S. as a child. African-Americans beat her for having pink skin and silver eyes. Whites beat her for "looking Jewish" and having black and curly hair along with Mongolian features, supposedly inherited from the Khazars and the peoples of the Silk Road. And, gee, nobody beat her for looking like my mother. When she was ten in the fifth grade, she asked a fellow student, "Do I look Jewish?"

The student replied, "You got the map of Jerusalem printed on your face."

On and on, mom would talk to me, and each time, there was another tale of how she played with neighbor kids and their German mothers would box her ears and call her epithets with the word "Jew" in them. The stereotype is of anyone from a Mediterranean country or the Caucasus Mountains who happens to have the profile of King Sargon of Babylon as his mask portrayed thousands of years ago, or a Sicilian profile with fair skin, light eyes, and dark hair. So why is it important?

What's not symmetrical enough for you? Well neither was the profile of King Tut, or Pharaoh Ramses, (may his mummy rest in peace) and nobody puts his finger to his nose and curls it convexly, except in a 1971 "All in the Family" episode followed by familiar canned laughter.

My early childhood experienced World War II, in Brooklyn. We lived in a four-family house near Kings Highway. Between the ages of three and five, not only did mom tell me about the holocaust in Europe, because I was born in 1941, but she would rock me in her arms when I was three, sweating in anxiety, as she sang to me about the bombs that were coming to fall on New York pretty soon. There were lights out air raid drills, and always she told me the bombs were coming to fall, and they never did.

The sweating, the anxiety was there anyway, almost as if they had come. Then she'd tell me about how the Irish and German Americans used to beat her for looking Jewish in the neighborhoods. She grew up (aged 10 to 14) during World War One. The street we lived on had been mostly Jewish on one side and partly southern Italian on the other, and almost never the twain met or spoke to one another.

Mom was a battered wife. Not only did I experience the holocaust from her stories, but the battles inside my home. My father, age 47 when I was born, and my brother, 13 years older than I, beat mom. There were terrible fights. I hid in my room and drew cartoons of them fighting.

One day my father smashed my piano and violin and all my birthday toys because I kicked him out of the bed I slept in with my mother when he tried to enter the bed in the middle of the night to have sex with my mother.

I was nine, and I told him to get out. He slept in the room next door in twin beds with my older brother in the room. Men with men, women with women, throughout my parent's marriage … and he beat her. And she told me about how he beat her when she came home from the hospital with me a week old, and he punched her in the chest, and I fell from her arms into the snow. She had told him to hurry up and take the baby's picture because I was turning blue from the cold wind and snow.

My father always smashed things with hammers and axes. I was afraid someday he'd get me and kill me. Mom told me how much she worried, about everything, and most of all how awful it was to be Jewish and be beaten for looking Jewish. As I grew up, I began to look in the mirror and wonder whether I looked Jewish. I had a "Caspian Sea Nose."

My cousins told me "I looked very Semitic." So I began to make myself up to look like an ancient Egyptian, eye makeup, black wig or hair tint, and costume. As I grew into a teenager, I took up the Turkish Belly dance, the Egyptian cane dance, the Moroccan dance, and the Zamba-Mora, a mixture of Flamenco and Moorish. My ballet lessons started at the age of five. By the age of eleven I danced on point—(toe).

At nine I gave a performance in ballet, a solo on the stage at my elementary school. At seven I started violin lessons and at nine, piano lessons. Music became my life. At thirteen I added voice lessons. I went on to graduate from college as a creative writing major, fine art minor, with second minors in psychology and anthropology. I was into ethnomusicology and linguistics. My hobby was astronomy and illustration … writing poetry, novels.

Then, at 22, I took a train back from a vacation in Asbury Park, returning to New York. I was married at the time, to a non-Jew. It was 1964, and the movie, *Cleopatra* was all over town. I had tinted my hair black; made my eyes up to look Egyptian, and thought I looked like Liz Taylor when I gazed back at myself in the mirror. In August of 1964 I was married, two months pregnant, and then my self-image melted.

A man, who I call the neo-Nazi, told me not to cross between cars while the train was in motion until the train stopped in Elizabeth, New Jersey. He wasn't the conductor. He was a passenger with his wife. I couldn't understand why he would order me to "wait 'till the train stopped in Elizabeth." I told him I was pregnant and returning from the john, and needed to get back to my seat or my husband and mother riding in the next car would think I became ill in the bathroom. He ignored me.

So I passed in front of him to return to my seat. I didn't brush him or touch his luggage or anything. There was no conductor around, and normally the right procedure is when you walk from one train car to the next to use the bathroom, it's regular procedure to walk back to your seat in the next car by opening and closing the easily sliding doors.

There were no train rules broken, of course. Because I didn't defer and defied his command, by walking past him to reach the next car and return silently to my seat and husband, he grabbed my head in a vise-like grip with his hand and knee, squeezed, trying to crush my head between his knee and the wall of the train causing me great pain in the skull, and beat the hell out of me by squeezing my head. The pain of my head being squeezed first between his large hands and then between his knees was unbearable.

Then he held me so I couldn't move and kicked me hard at the base of the spine while he yelled, "you dirty Jew." I went flying forward into the next car while his wife eyed my wedding ring as I faced her for a moment, and quietly smirked, "let her go, dear."

She had the sweetest controlled voice as she looked up at me behind the fishnet veil of her pillbox hat. The two reminded me of the painting, "Gothic American." He was bald, black hair around the rim of his ears, staring black eyes, pale skin. She looked the same with curled brown hair and wrinkles above her thin lips. The words, "dirty Jew," rang in my head. I walked back to my seat two cars down and never said a word to my husband or mother.

My husband would have returned and started a fight. My mother had just gotten out of the hospital and was recuperating. For the next twenty years I never said a word … to anyone. My fear of being Jewish went inward and increased. When I wrote about my experience, some women accused me of being "a man-hater."

The next day I stopped trying to look like Elizabeth Taylor in *Cleopatra*. I bleached the black tint out of my brown hair and made it bright red. With the freckles and hazel green eyes, I announced to the mirror that I now looked Welsh. Funny, how nobody noticed my convex nose, I surmised, when my hair was medium ash blonde or Killarney russet.

A few times during my teenage years in Brooklyn, some Puerto Ricans asked me whether I were Scottish or Irish. One black man tried to strangle me without asking what I was first. He only asked where my money was. A white man asked me once where the synagogue was, but I remember seeing him on TV as one of the skinheads taken into custody.

He was teasing me. First he asked me whether I needed help crossing the street and called me old lady. When I told him my age as if to say, I'm not that old, he brought up the Jewish lady part, emphatically with fury and frustration.

I was over age 60-something then and turned around and told him this face is what Mediterranean people look like. At that point in a public street in a Mexican area of San Diego, I was disgusted and just tired of people asking me where I'm from and what I am. Every time I opened my mouth I was asked when I had come from New York. In one city, I walked into a seminar in Jewish history and heard that the professor had received death threats when he was appointed chairman of the Jewish Studies department that sponsored the free seminars at a university open to the public.

Most people who showed up were over age sixty and a few history students. So much for freedom of speech in a state university hall, it seems. The next lecture I went to was on quilting. The teacher never got any threats teaching crafts. All I went there for was to make a friend and find some place to belong. I still don't belong anywhere and have not yet made an attempt to make friends, although I want to. It became harder to find friends after age sixty-three, and I never learned to drive—too scared to take tests anymore.

It's more than forty years since I left Brooklyn. Why is it so important?

I seldom speak in public, but talk to my video camera frequently. Then I let the videos become available to individuals seeking information.

I've become a recluse to have some semblance of serenity. Better to be alone than to be 'pecked.' On the Internet people stop asking about my New York accent online. The silence of e-mail distracts them from even wanting to know. Interestingly enough, the man who beat me never bothered to ask first whether I was Jewish, Greek, or Armenian, or any other Eastern Mediterranean national or descended from, thereof, because we all look alike to him, but he singled out "Jew" and beat me for looking Jewish. I am an American with parents born in New York State.

What is Jewish supposed to look like, an Assyrian king of 3,500 years ago? Why do most Assyrian Christians look so much like me? With whom does my DNA cluster? Why can't we all accept one another's diversity without asking, without making it so important to know what someone's core identity is in privacy. I'm not your egg donor, so why ask? Nearly each time I open my mouth someone asks me when I left New York. I've been out of New York since 1965.

The man on the train who beat me didn't ask my name or look to see whether I wore a cross or a star or anything else. For a moment I wanted to say, "I'm Maltese. This is the face of Malta, or Naples, or Istanbul, or Crete." Perhaps my 38 college units in anthropology would have come in handy at that moment. But I said nothing for decades after that event.

So scared was my mother of being Jewish that she first joined the Dutch reformed Protestant church in Brooklyn and took me there when I was nine. We landed in the Unitarian church for decades. I also went to many other churches in the neighborhood. At the Catholic Church, the nun once said to me, "I don't think you're Catholic. You look Jewish. What's your name?" I replied, "Angelica," because we lived near an Italian neighborhood, and I used to ask my Christian friends to donate their old rosaries to me because I collected them for those who needed them.

I learned my "hail Mary's" and pinned up all the rosaries in our basement where I lit a candle on Shabbat and prayed in Hebrew and in English, both the Catholic "hail Mary's" and the Jewish Sabbath blessing prayer every Friday night. I spoke to Jesus and anyone else listening and asked a lot of philosophical questions, and wrote a book of prayers when I was nearly twelve.

Then I started reading Tibetan Buddhism and all about reincarnation from other religions, including the Eastern religions. I saw religion as links on a chain knowing we all come from and go to the same place.

A loving God would not have created people in the first place unless he, she, or it, the Creator or designer sent us to the same place equally and took us from that place to be born again and again. I wondered who wrote the Bible with all those inconsistencies and contradictions, but thought it was great to have all that control over people who really would do you wrong, and freedom to choose for all the people seeking for the highest right for the good of all.

I ended up marrying an Arab Sheik at 21. When I was pregnant, he beat the hell out of me. The marriage ended when I became a battered wife, and he took my two children to Syria where his mother and six brothers reared them after he divorced me and took away all the money in the bank, my furniture, and threw me out into the street after more than 6 years of marriage. At 33 I married a Protestant man, American, half German, half English. We are now married more than 30 years. I can't think of anyone who loves me, except my cat.

He used to beat me too, but far less than the Sheik, mostly more verbally, but twice a year physically, but now he's only verbally abusive and beats me only once a year if he can catch me when I run from him. He beats me only when we are moving from one house to another, and he's stressed. He has intermittent explosive disorder to some degree and explodes when he doesn't get his way, like when he wanted some old bookcases for fifty dollars, and I wanted something new.

I'm still married to him. He never reads what I write, and I write under different names. When he quiets down, he's back to his old withdrawn cold fish self just like daddy. We have not shared the same room for almost 30 years, his choice first, not mine, but now his snoring is loud enough to cause me insomnia. I've been celibate since 1976. He has no affection for me, but I don't have to pay rent. That's great as I don't have an income although I'd love an income.

When I think about it, I surmise on the MBTI ® I'm an INFP. A wife isn't supposed to complain about her cold-fish husband according to etiquette, but like my mother and women generations before her, I'm a low self-esteem, low confidence woman who can't take care of herself married to a man who can't take care of a wife. He's a commanding, bullying, whining and volcanic ISFJ with low serotonin levels, high narcissism and worry about self image, and I'm financially dependent upon him in my old age and nearly penniless compared to most other women with graduate school liberal arts educations. I'm shy, frightened, old, and spent, but I like the free rent, the backyard, and my doggies who do show me affection by wagging their tails when I give them their food and a hug. So I don't plan to budge unless I'm thrown to the curb. Then I will be a homeless old woman with on and off agoraphobia and panic disorder.

My husbands became abusive dads to me, just like my own dad, but since my present husband abuses me far less than the first husband did, I'll stay as long as there's money to pay the taxes on the house and keep food in the fridge.

I married my first husband at 21, the Sheik because I thought in a previous life, I had come from Egypt or Syria, but digging deeper, I found at that at 13 I was secretly in love with a Syrian Jewish boy in my class because he was rich, lived in a private house on Ocean Parkway, and was handsome.

A clique of Syrian Jewish girls said I could join their 8th grade sorority if I took all my clothes off in front of them and let their 6-year old brother feel me up. Wanting so bad to join their clique, I went into the closet and took off all my clothes. The girls grabbed my clothes, tossed them over my head, playing monkey in the middle, and humiliated me.

Then they pushed me out of their house and into the gutter with me barely missing the path of an oncoming car by inches. I was totally intimidated and humiliated. Thereafter, I never had a friend for years.

Later, I tried making friends with a Jewish girl. She was rich, an Ashkenazi, and became my best friend. But she betrayed me like the others. When I confided in her, making her like a sister, that my mom was arrested for shoplifting and I was so shocked, she turned around and made up a lie that I had stolen her empty purse. Her mother called my brother and screamed about my mother being a shoplifter. She never knew my mother. I didn't take her purse and never would have thought such thoughts.

All I wanted to be is accepted by the rich, or those richer than I was. Her father practiced law. Mine was a janitor and 8th-grade dropout, born in 1894 in New York. She kept asking me to return the purse. I kept asking why she'd make up such as story and then tell her mother about my mother, or why her mother would call my older brother and rub his nose in the dirt that my mother was arrested for shoplifting, when I had told her daughter this in confidence as my best friend.

Needless to say, I have no friends today, no living relatives beyond my distant children that I know of, and a husband who puts me down verbally, teases me, and sometimes batters me. People seem to have betrayed me a lot. And yet, I still hope someday I'll find a friend.

I'm no longer as 'sociophobic' as in my twenties. But I still fear people, especially when total strangers drop a heavy arm on my shoulder and start a conversation when meeting me for the first time. Nor do I walk through life totally alone any more. I can choose joining associations or meditating in isolation, usually home-based. I spend many days reading and writing or walking through the zoo.

One freedom I cherish. It's to belong to several religions at one time and to attend all the churches, synagogues, or other houses of worship that I want—usually the Unitarian. I go to Christian churches on Christian holidays and to Jewish synagogues on Jewish holidays.

I want my freedom to choose any religion anytime and to attend any celebration of life. I cherish this freedom because I believe God is love and that we all come from and go to the same place. No creator creates any intelligent being unequal to any other intelligent being on any universe. And our companion pets come with us into eternity and give us comfort.

For a decade I was housebound with agoraphobia and panic between age 23 and 33. It burned itself out without any treatment, as I was penniless. Today, I have two computers, a paid-off home, and it's all his. I'm still too scared to tell anyone I'm Jewish, except other Jews. I belong to the Unitarian church, and I still celebrate, alone, the Jewish holidays.

My two children are devout Muslims, still trying to convert me to Islam and talking about Jews at the same time, warning me not to tell their friends that I'm Jewish. I smile to their face. I'm forbidden to tell my grandchildren my religion. What religion? I'm one with the universe because we all come from and go back to the exact same place. I'll read the book or Bible of any religion and contemplate all the good points.

Why am I scared to be Jewish? The Skinheads and Neo Nazis are all over this town. I am respected in the Unitarian church. I give donations to the Jewish organizations. Secretly, I sneak off to "Chabad" and dance with the Hasidim, clapping my hands in joy. For an hour it feels like I have a loving daddy there smiling, alive with fervor, and yet peaceful. Maybe in real life women are not as equal in his family. I don't know. Each person is different. Maybe women at home are treated as an equal. I won't judge. I only want to enjoy the happiness for that moment in time ... that I am blessed by someone who for that hour is like real family.

That's why I write books on how to write family history newsletters. In real life, nobody really calls or visits that were once part of my parent's family—the children and descendants of people related to my parents. You ask, why don't I write to them? I did for a time, but they didn't like some of the plays I wrote and stopped writing. No, the plays did not name them or their city.

And what about my children and children in law? They are devout Muslims, popular physicians in America that phone me on my birthday and mother's day to say hello. They ask, "How are you?" I say, "Great." And they reply that they are doing fine, are financially okay, and are popular physicians. The only conversational 'object' I lack are platonic friends and companions. I have no friends. I really am afraid that if I make close friends with a woman that she'll take my present husband away.

I am not physically able to compete with another woman for the financial support my husband gives me—the free room and utilities. If only my past female friends didn't betray me, I think. Yet I am open to making new friends that don't require that I do what I cannot do—lend them money.

Many have asked in the past. On the allowance for food my husband gives me each week, there's no way I can spare money to lend to friends. Perhaps someday friends that don't ask me to lend them money will come along, and perhaps female friends that don't try to take my husband away also will appear.

It would be nice to find friends that are not so needy for my only means of financial support. What I seek from friends is to listen to what works for them spiritually. Perhaps I can find friends that already have love, companionship, and enough money. I need to feel safe around others.

It's good to know that it is okay to practice any religion or no religion as long as one's beliefs or conclusions are about lessening stress, resolving conflicts, doing good, repairing, healing, or healthy attitudes. I already have closure. What I need now is stress reduction and fun. I need to learn how to laugh more. It's healthy. I can laugh at myself. What else can I laugh at that's not about putting people down?

During Christmas week I'm in a wide variety of churches listening to the fine carols and playing them on my organ in a celebration of life. And I still belly dance to Middle Eastern music when I'm alone at home.

I love all peoples and cherish their music as a divine gift to humankind. In soothing music from all cultures I find the harmony and serenity of healing. On Rosh Hashanah, Yom Kippur and Passover, I go to various synagogues. On Easter, I enjoy a Greek Orthodox, Episcopal, or Roman Catholic Mass because I can meditate and watch the flickering candles that lessen stress for me. I love listening to the melody of the hymns. Music is healing.

My mother always scared the living daylights out of me by saying that someday there's going to be another holocaust right here in America and they'll get me if I tell anyone I'm Jewish. I really don't know when or if that might happen. I pray not. I cherish the freedom of religion and the separation of church and state.

I'm always hiding my face with my hands, scared to panic that someone will see my Hittite, Roman nose and automatically react with violence because everyone knows what a "Jewish nose" is supposed to look like, but few know what a Persian, Armenian, or Roman nose is supposed to be. The Hittite nose is a feature native to Anatolia, Syria, and Northern Iraq in Neolithic times.

There's no such protuberance as a "Jewish nose" any more than there's something called a "Christian nose" or a "Buddhist nose." A convex nose is the result of a round headed parent marrying a long-headed parent in any country.

The child born of a parent with the genes for at least 33 to 50 percent round, short-headedness and a parent with the genes for at least 33 to 50 percent of long, low-skulled heads as seen in some Northern and Southern European countries, the Middle East, or Persia will create a child with a different type of skull—flat in the back (occiput) with a long, convex nose.

That child can come from any country. You see this type frequently in Switzerland, Austria, Italy, France, the Adriatic, Turkey, Iraq, Syria, the Balkans, and anywhere else that short-headed people have married long-headed people of any religion or nation. In races other than Caucasian, you get the same result: short heads married to long heads beget children with large, convex noses and flat backs of the heads (occiputs) much of the time.

Ask someone to draw a Jewish nose and you get a number '6'. Ask someone to draw a Roman nose—an ancient one of an aristocrat—and they are not sure or they draw the letter 'L.' The whole picture in people's minds is built on years of cartoon caricature stereotypes and models used for painting. The painting of the 14th century poet, Dante Alleghieri shows the North Italian poet from Florence, a devout Catholic with a most extreme convex nose. Nobody cares because he's an Italian Catholic. If he were Jewish, painters would have used him in Renaissance paintings to depict famous Biblical Jews.

The reason I'm alluding to Dante is because I'm tired of total strangers walking up to me at bus benches telling me I'm Jewish. They don't even ask.

It has nothing to do with being Jewish. It has all to do with being intimidated and humiliated—not because the convex nose is so fervently associated with a consciousness of being Jewish, but with a myth that if you have a convex nose, you must be Jewish, and therefore treated like Jews had been treated in the days of the Venice ghetto.

And the stereotype can reinforce sociophobia in people vulnerable to panic disorder. Imagine what it feels like when I sit in a Christian church wondering whether anyone is looking at my nose or the scar on my face. I couldn't care less about the scar.

It's the shape of my nose that they are looking at. They are probably wondering what I'm doing in their church. It's all right, I tell myself, to look as I do. I don't need a plastic surgeon to give me back my self-confidence, to shorten my nose, or to remove a scar already partly hidden in my old-age wrinkles.

Ladies pushing 70 with white hair are so invisible anyway, I surmise, that it isn't necessary to spend money on my face and hair. Better I spend it on having fun and visiting the seashore, several hours away by train. Lord, it feels so great to be invisible and not singled out in a public place such as a church, theatre, or lecture hall.

Taking away one's freedom of worship is akin to being told you have the wrong country's nose and that a surgeon must take off what identifies you. It's like being told that thousands of years ago an ancestor came from a certain place and that has to be corrected. A plastic surgeon once said he'd take the hump off my nose, but what's the point? I don't need symmetry to feel beautiful on the outside or inside. I need the experience of joyful song. I hope no more mayhem will happen, hope so much that I pray tensely with my eyelids squeezed shut.

The only thing I can do about it is to try to make the world a kinder and gentler place, being the idealist that I am as I do my housewifely crafts and write a novel a year to keep active. I go to a wide variety of churches and hold my head up high, and I go to the synagogue and hold my head up high, and I don't want anybody calling me ethnic names or hating me because my great-great grandparents practiced a particular religion in a country I've never seen.

We all have a right to follow more than one religion and have fun exploring the different aspects. I'm reading Mary Baker Eddy's book, and I'm enjoying Christian Science. I also like Science of Mind and Religious Science and Unity and all the new age churches and painting mandalas and Tibetan Buddhist philosophy and meditation for a few minutes at home for peace's sake.

My favorite author is Ray Bradbury. We all see things, not the way they are, but the way we are. A hate crime doesn't have to play on stage where observers can distance themselves. Fear doesn't have to take top billing publicly; it can be internal.

When will it be okay anywhere in the world to follow your spiritual meditations privately and not be chastised publicly for your symmetry or hue?

How are we all doing with visual shorthand? I have not "gotten a life." Instead, I've learned to forgive others and myself. Why would a nice, Jewish girl from Coney Island marry an Arab Sheik **and live disguised as an Arab housewife in a Jewish section of Brooklyn for nearly seven years**? Maybe because we all come from and go to the same place or maybe because in a former life I was both, maybe I'm looking for something beyond a core identity, or maybe I just want a connection to everyone else in the world, but on a higher plane that reaches beyond territory and tribe to universal archetypes.

After all, you get to the universal only through the concrete details with which we all identify across cultures. Everyone on the planet is connected by a common ancestor. I'm connected to the three fellows who lived somewhere in the Middle East 7,800 years ago, the woman who lived in Europe 20,000 years ago, and the rest who left the Fertile Crescent, Central Asia, Africa, or India between 60,000 and 30,000 years ago for better campgrounds.

They are all connected to me by my DNA and love of art, music, and writing. Family stories are *evidence* of who we are. 'Salable' life stories usually are launched in the media—the major national press of credible repute—before they are produced as a video or movie and published as a book. Personal histories, like corporate histories may end up as time capsules on disk and on Web sites as video and audio documentaries or in books.

4

Becoming Agoraphobic

Does Marriage or Genes Most Influence the Persistence of Agoraphobia?

So which situation is the schlemiel or the schlemazel here—genes, early childhood attitudes, environment, or being intimidated and controlled by an angry partner in a marriage? Does there really have to be one cause of panic disorder?" No.

Everything works together. But it's the fact that you or I have inherited a short copy or 'version' of the 5-HTTP gene that may be responsible for you or me not being able to walk out of a marriage where you are bullied. If your body isn't letting you find a secure way to earn an income over many decades, look to electrical/chemical hyperactivity in your brain's fear center.

What's Arab-Jewish intermarriage like? "It's reaching for Rajasthan from Litvakistan through a Coney Island Kasha Knish stand. Why live disguised seven years as an Arab housewife in an Orthodox Jewish Neighborhood in Brooklyn of the early sixties to start a visual anthropology-through-journalism research career? What did I find out that's universal?" (Note all names and places have been changed for privacy in this book.)

Winter, 1941 Brooklyn New York

"Poland is for Poles, not for Jews," the man in the street yelled to my grandfather in Bialystock. "If I share a percentage of my genes with other Semites such as you," my grandfather said to the Arab Muslim and Arab Christian men in New York, then why can't I live in the Middle East and be accepted as one of you?"

"You're different genetically, with all those freckles and blue eyes and red hair" the Arab answered. "How's that, like you don't have as many Roman and Greek genes among those Semitic ones as I might have German, Polish or Sorb genes mixed with my Middle Eastern ones?" He looked at grandpa. "But I have black hair and a light brown skin, and you're white."

Grandpa smiled, "And half the people in Lebanon are white with brown hair and hazel eyes, like the rest of my family." The Arab grinned, "Maybe that's why all of us are now living here in New York. Do you think Jesus looked Jewish or Arab?" Grandpa scowled over his shoulder in a voice dark as lava. "He probably looked Roman enough to end up in the Vatican."

The only tone that separates the music of the Arab from Jewish Klezmer music of Eastern Europe is the 'G' note on an instrument string. My life is about growing up Jewish secular, marrying an Arab Muslim, his divorcing me, taking our two children and all money and community property, leaving me bare and poor as I was born, and searching for identity in the healing sound of music and writing. I begin again with only a pitch of tone separating me between the worlds of the Hassid and the worlds of the Arab.

That's why I wrote this memoir: growing up in disguise as an Arab housewife in a Jewish world of Bensonhurst in Brooklyn, New York. I'm a Polish Jew, but why don't I look Polish? Why do I look Arab? I'm supposed to look just like another Pole if what the Arabs say, that Polish Jews are mostly Polish, but I look Arab. Could my ancestry really be mostly from a common ancestor in the Middle East thousands of years ago?

Or am I another daughter of the Sorbs, the Lusatians of East Germany and Western Poland whose ancestors converted to Judaism in medieval times? If so, then why do I look as if I just stepped out of ancient Babylon or Lebanon? Where do I belong, my friends? For seven years I lived in disguise dressed as an Arab woman, eating, speaking, living, and going about my business as an Arab housewife in the early 1960s, married to an Arab Muslim—living in the center of a Jewish world in Bensonhurst in Brooklyn.

I'm an American Hasidic Polish Jew living a secular life of searching for a faith in which men and women are treated equally in eternity regardless of what universe they come from. I'm tired of the takeaway man. Love can never be taken away. Yet that all is what we perceive has been taken away. Even the universe has a life span. But love is forever. Is love and consciousness one super intelligence that uses love to make sure life will never be contained from inhabiting all the dimensions of all the parallel universes? If so, why can't we feel love and peace directed toward us in the home, let alone in the public world?

Some people do. Wonderful. How do I find it? By being a loving person even when not loved? Great idea. If the government didn't love all of us, there wouldn't be social security for those of us whose only incomes are social security.

Or are politics and constitutions forms of love? Did Thomas Jefferson and friends so love the world that he made sure his peers wrote a constitution that would guarantee us a Bill of Human rights—or just bills?

Why did I make visual anthropology part of my life as a long reading list? To see how the other side feels and receives? Was it worth it? Decide for yourself. In doing so, I lost my two children, all community property, all money in the bank, and when he divorced me, I re-entered the world bare as I was born, with twenty-eight cents to my name, and no living relatives who knew me or cared.

Then, when my children grew up and returned, as devout Muslims and Arabs, they forbid me to tell my grandchildren that my ancestry was Jewish. Being the adult child of a Jewish mother and an Arab Muslim father (from Syria) is unique, but the intermarriage rate is on the rise. How do the children feel? Is it a social stigma?

We travel in different worlds, social circles, customs, celebrations, yet we come from the same common ancestor, or do we? And does anybody out there care? As a visual anthropologist, I wanted to see how the other side lived. Now, in my mid-sixties, I am excruciatingly alone, my only solace two large dogs and two cats, and days filled with writing and art and anthropology. What's it like to be the child of Arab and Jewish parents? Although there are Jewish women in Israel who have married Palestinian Arab men and live in Arab villages with their children, how do they feel once their children are grown, they are old like me, and perhaps widowed like me from their Arab husbands? Whom do they remarry?

Do they return to Judaism or turn to Christianity or remain in the Muslim villages? What happens to them in Israel? What about those marriages in America? Here's my own story, set in Brooklyn, New York in an apartment where everyone was pious, Hasidic Jews from Eastern Europe, and I was the only Hasidic Polish Jewish girl whose parents broke away from orthodox parents of their own, became secular, and by my generation of the 1950s, somehow set me spinning into choosing a mate who was 'different.' I married an Arab Muslim from Syria. After six and a half years of marriage, he divorced me. Here is my story.

You can figure out why I dared to marry outside my own religion. It goes beyond the fact that I lived in a house of domestic violence. My mom was a battered wife. The moral of the story is that no matter how far I reached to marry a man who wouldn't batter me the way my dad battered my mom, I married a man exactly like my dad. Even though my dad was a Polish Jew and I married an Arab Muslim to reach out for something different, I ended up just as much of a battered wife as my own mother was.

The point is that it doesn't matter what ethnic group your husband is. If he has an explosive temper and hits you, he could be any ethnicity or religion. I struggled with the decision about the clash of cultures. Sure, it's better to marry someone from your own background, but what if the genes are too close or too inbred in your ethnic group? All I wanted was to marry a man in whose presence I could feel safe at all times. I wanted a husband and family in whose presence I could go to sleep at night and know I would awake in the morning alive. Here's my story.

Slovenly dressed, whippet-wiry Meyer tried to adjust the lens on his box camera. Snow flurries slashed his face with a thousand thongs, covering his white hair and long beard as his breath steamed into the morning frost of West First Street.

Tsipke, his wife, carried in one arm her pink-blanketed two-week old daughter, me, the half-Jewish girl. In her other arm she tried to balance a bouquet of deep, red American Beauty roses. The blanket kept blowing over the baby's face as Tsipke fidgeted to straighten it. A nerve-shattering cry pierced the wind.

"Hurry and take the picture. The baby's turning blue." Tsipke shouted at Meyer. And the shouts seemed to be coming from a horde of crones, screaming together in fury, cutting him to pieces. All he saw was the open mouth of his wife, Tsipke, the Jewish girl he married in 1926. Her voice became an indistinguishable roar of needy demand as loud as the wind.

Again, Meyer tried to focus the lens of his camera. For a moment Tsipke tried to smile and look into the camera.

They stood just outside their four-family brick house. From inside echoes of Bach pealed through the tiny apartment, as if coming from the tin-can sound of an old phonograph. And as a mighty fugue ravaged the ten by ten rooms, the subway elevator line grinded by, drowning out the music.

"The baby is freezing', you jerk."

"Shut up! Damn it. I'm trying to keep the lens from getting wet."

"Hurry up, you neurotic. She can't breathe."

Tsipke yelled again, her voice a compelling tattoo. Then Meyer's temper cracked, and he let fly with a right hook to her left chest. The baby slid from the blanket into the soft snow drift. Meyer couldn't stop punching his wife. Her worry about health would always be met with punches, until her body couldn't take one more punch.

The American beauty roses scattered on the snow and formed a collage against the shiny black of the baby's hair. I am that dark-haired baby now white-haired, with the shining Topaz-green eyes.

◆   ◆   ◆

5

Winter 1950 Same Brooklyn Apartment

I squirmed awake next to my mother in the rutted double bed in which we both slept. Meyer, in the next bedroom slept in twin beds with his 22-year old son. It was three in the morning. Outside the window the sound of the grinding subway never ceased. Only the pouring rain soothed the screeching of the cars on the track as they turned the corner on their way to Coney Island.

"Remember when we played Suffering'? And I'd rub your belly, and your doll would be delivered like a baby?" Tsipke laughed and grunted her hacking cigarette cough.

Mom rolled over, pulling my mass of dark hair from my eyes. "I'm sick of hearing about your lousy sex life. Geez. Quit harping. I don't want to hear any more of it."

"You're nine today. You gotta know."

The radiator had dried out the air in the room. My mouth and nose felt paper-thin and raw as I trembled. Meyer tiptoed out of his bedroom and crawled into bed with his wife.

"What the hell are you doing here?" I provoked him.

Meyer took off his pajamas and climbed into bed to have sex with his wife.

"Get the hell outta here, you son of a bitch."

"You kicking' me out?" Meyer hesitated for a moment.

"The kid said she had a 130 I.Q." Tsipke interrupted.

"Shut up, you tramp."

"Don't call me a tramp."

"Better you should be crippled. You should have been born a boy. I'll kill you, you piece of garbage."

Meyer hurried his pajamas back on and stormed out looking for something to smash. He found a hammer in the living room and began to smash all the keys on my piano. My birthday. I had almost forgotten.

Tsipke had saved seventy-five dollars from the three dollars a day Meyer gave her and bought me a used upright for my ninth birthday. When Meyer finished smashing the piano keys, he went for the violin that Tsipke gave me for last year's birthday.

The violin had been bought in 1936 for brother's seventh birthday. After a year or two of lessons, he gave it up. For years it had stood among Benjamin's undusted toys, forgotten in the cellar.

Meyer put his foot through the violin. Finally, he grabbed my new puppy and held its belly against the hot radiator pipe in the bathroom until it stopped whimpering.

I looked in on mother, but Tsipke didn't move or respond to my presence. She just lied there, staring at the ceiling, and I always felt that long ago she had given up all effort. I would never give up trying to find a life, an identity, a self, or a sense of belonging. I ran into the living room.

"Not my birthday presents. Don't smash my presents." I cried.

The louder the sounds of her voice grew the more terrified and angry Meyer became. He began to chase me around the apartment waving the hammer over his head like a madman.

"If I catch you, I'll cripple you." Heads will roll before you'll become a tramp." He went for the ax in his private closet, putting the hammer away. I scampered under a table and crouched there, sobbing.

"I'm sorry. I'm sorry, daddy."

"Better you should be crippled than to be born a girl and make trouble for me."

"I should have flushed her out into the bay with the condom. Better she wasn't made or born," Meyer raged.

"If I have to get up for a cigarette. Damn, those cigarettes are killing me. But you two fighting are driving me to smoke."

At last Tsipke hurried into the kitchen and lit a cigarette, making the motions of heating up water for coffee. "Leave the kid alone."

Meyer, now angry with Tsipke, took a swing at me with the hammer, and missed. I darted cut of the kitchen and dashed out the front door in the living room, down the apartment steps, and then down the cellar steps. In the darkness, Meyer chased his daughter, gaining on me as I disappeared into the basement.

A partially filled coal bin accepted my body. Inside the old barrel the dark space felt cool, moldy, and damp as I covered myself with coal. Meyer looked around for a few seconds, wild-eyed, wiping the beaded sweat on his upper lip on his pajama sleeve. "If I catch you, I'll kill you."

From between the wide slats of the coal bin I watched as he swung his hammer overhead. As he passed a work table, Meyer slapped an ax against his thigh a couple of times. Then he sighed and left it on the table. Finally, exhausted, he plodded up the wooden stairs.

The apartment door closed with a bang. No sooner did Meyer stalk into the kitchen then Tsipke, in her best shrill, let him have her words as if they were machine gun bullets.

"No sooner did I put the baby on your lap then you told me to take her off because she gave you an erection."

"You keep hounding me just because your step father came into your room to have sex with you when you went to visit your mother."

"He's your rich brother. Besides I threw him out, but you don't see him grabbing an ax and a hammer."

"Girls only make trouble. You know how many times I asked the doctor to check to make sure-maybe he made a mistake-maybe she was a boy?"

"Is that why you never held a conversation with your daughter or even smiled at her? Not once in your whole life did you ever talk to the kid straight."

"What about you going into your son's room to massage his feet ever' morning and comb his hair?

"I'm a mother."

"He's twenty-two. He says you're overbearing."

"I'm going back to bed."

"Where is she?"

"In the cellar again. Let her rot in hell down there."

Meyer staggered back to bed. Tsipke spent the rest of the night smoking cigarettes and reading old newspapers.

In the morning I peeked out of the basement window and scratched off some of the frost. I watched father go off to work, walking toward the subway station. Then I climbed the stairs back up to her world and knocked on my family's door. Tsipke wore the same stained and disheveled flannel housedress she wore the day before. But it covered her five-foot tall, 250-pound rotundity well, her flapping ham-hock upper arms and her la banza belly.

Benjamin, my older brother by fourteen years had a short temper.

"Benjamin had a fight with me over you making too much noise," Mom told me when I came home from school.

"And he broke a lamp over my arm. But I dared him to do it."

"Does daddy know?"

"I had to tell him. So now he smashed your brother's typewriter just before his first year law school exam."

"I'm too tired to go to school today." I shuffled into the foyer, passing the dead canary in the green bird cage.

"It caught a virus. You'll have to take it down to the garbage cans."

"Oh, no. Well, it will reincarnate as something else." I ran into the bedroom.

"Listen, you little mouse. Want to go shopping?" Tsipke went back to frying eggs and put down a heel of rye bread for me and some hot cocoa and sugared corn flakes. The whole kitchen smelled of hot chocolate with cinnamon. Even at nine, I worried about being stuffed with so much sugar that I shook from hypoglycemia tremors. Panic disorder haunted me most of my life.

The subway let off the two of us near Borough Hall and Fulton St. We walked to Mays and Lane Bryant to look at the dresses for larger women. I was even skinnier than Meyer. From the back the two of us looked like a skinny midget Abbott and a balloon of Costello. Kids in my fourth grade class on West First Street and Avenue "P" in Brooklyn called me skinny malink. Years later, I learned malinka in Polish meant something like 'darling'.

Mom and I walked through May's department store looking at the baubles and silken wisps of underwear, the sweet, sickly scent of cheap cologne, and the boxes of face powder.

On her way Tsipke shoplifted white-pink lipsticks, rhinestone broaches, clip-on earrings, negligees in size 34-which could never fit her Reubenesque rotundity, and tiny training bras size 32 AAA. When no one WAS looking in the ladies room, she'd stuff clothing into her incontinence panties.

"I don't want any of the beads or perfume," I whispered from the next toilet stall. "They're cursed. You'll get bad luck."

Tsipke banged the metal wall of the cubicle. "Your father only gives me chickenfeed. How else can I live?"

"I don't want to wear that crap." She would always lay a curled-smoke curse on me like a Coney Island 'fot' when I misbehaved, and then I'd punish myself by having an accident. I had set it up unconsciously to get rid of the tension.

Laying the fear on me with the palms caused the anxiety, and later I had to get relief by getting hurt, getting the accident over with. I realized that by the time I became a teenager. At nine, there was only the curse, and the punishment I inflicted on myself fired from deep within me like a salty cold well to keep my sensibilities.

"Here, stuff this nightgown in your panties."

"No! I won't."

Tsipke dragged whining me into the dressing room with some of the items tucked inside of dresses because only three garments were allowed in the dressing rooms at one time. In front of the mirror Tsipke put on bras, slips, and clothing under her own clothes. She brought out the three garments she took into the fitting rooms.

"These dresses aren't the right size." Tsipke handed the two dresses over to the sales clerk. She waddled into the shoe department to buy I a pair of saddle shoes for school clothes. Mother and daughter sat down in the shoe department.

"Give me that skinny foot," said the salesman, trying to shove one of the new shoes on my dirt-caked foot.

"Leave me alone!" I shouted, storming out of the shoe section. I shouted the big four-letter word at him as I looked over my shoulder.

"That filthy kid," he stammered.

Tsipke caught up to her daughter in women's lingerie. "Horseface, why the hell did you say that?"

"He didn't have to call me skinny like in ugly."

"Why did you have to wear those old socks? You're beginning to stink just like your old man who's never taken a bath since he came out of World War One."

Later, riding home in the subway, I finished reading her two comic books, "The Vault of Horror" and "The Crypt of Terror" that Tsipke bought her in the candy store will her gill of chocolate ice cream to take home.

"Where's your old man, where's the bastard?"

"Probably at one of his flower shows."

"Some men come straight home after work. Meyer, he's got his flower shows. Did you know he caught VD when you're brother was five?"

"What's VD?"

"Got it from some whore, I betcha. He told me it came back from his World War One days. Thinks I've got my mamma's head."

"See this scar on my face?" I grimaced.

"So?"

"That's because you cursed me last year. Did you think your curse would give me eight stitches?"

"Where the hell is your old man? He's never home, the bastard."

"I told you that stuff you steal brings me bad luck. I always end up falling over fences at school and getting stitches."

"Shut up! The subway's crowded."

"Everybody in school calls me crazy. When I grow up nobody nice will marry me."

I sighed and pulled out her drawing pad and crayons from her shoulder bag. She began to draw a grotesque face with pointy fingers on her small art pad. The face is contorted with gaping month and reptilian.

"What kind of happy face is that?"

"I don't know. But it makes me happy to do it."

"Say, you're brother's taking you on a trip across the George Washington Bridge on Sunday."

That weekend Benjamin strolled with me along the pedestrian path. He stopped at the highest point on the bridge to gaze at the view. Suddenly Benjamin gave me a shove against the railing and then pulled me back before I could let out a wail.

"Stop fooling around. You've no right to scare me like that."

"Like what?" As always, he denied and began to sing. "Come, come my child, to the devil we must go."

He lifted me up to the railing and laughed. I lashed out, flailing, screaming in terror. Benjamin put me down harshly. "Oh, stop being a sissy, a baby, smartass."

"Why do you always do that to me?" I kicked the railing.

"'Cause you're my baby sister."

◆   ◆   ◆

6

Booklyn Junior High School Classroom, September 1955

I sat in the middle of the Syrian Jewish clique surrounded by tsetse Fly Arleen, Fatstummik Seeley, and Bee-eyed Busta. These were the nicknames I gave to the sorority, the clique of Aleppo's that filled up the ranks of my eighth-grade class. At twelve-and-a half, my seventy-five pound body was no match for the pubescent. The pale, freckled girl with the pony-tailed dark ash brown hair and Topaz-with-olive-green eyes.

I couldn't break into the Syrian clique no matter how hard I tried to join the Meghas or the Cheetahs junior high school sororities. Not unless I changed my last name.

Should I pick a Sephardic one and get into the clique of the Brooklyn rich few, or an Ashkenazi name at enter the clique of the uptown rich? Or perhaps grandma's Jewish name, and be on my own in a family that only wanted me to hide everything and reach for a rich husband from a poor neighborhood. Brother told me to forget the husband.

"You're too ugly to meet a good provider. So get your own career and make it as a stockbroker," he said at least once a day.

I wasn't what the clique wanted. Why would they let in an Ashkenazim girl, when they only wanted a girl from Aleppo, a Halebi. I wasn't a Syrian Jew; I wasn't a Portuguese Marrano from Belmonte, but I wanted to be just like them. I wanted to have a private house with a maid on Ocean Parkway, go to Florida for vacations, and have a rich, loving dad who owned his own profitable business have enough money to enjoy "the good life" and not beat me or threaten me or call me names.

I wanted a Syrian Jewish husband who was kind and had enough money to support me so I could spend my life taking art lessons and shopping for a living like I heard Syrian Jewish women do. Where did I hear that? From poor Eastern

European Jewish girls who lived in tiny apartments and sat out on their stoops on Saturday night and chatted about how the Syrian Jewish ladies got to own their own private houses, while we Polish American Jews still lived in tiny, fourth-floor walkup apartments. Will somebody rich and kind please marry me I hoped at age thirteen.

I had a Jewish, mother whose own mother came from Bessarabia, now in Moldova, and a Jewish father from Bialystock, Poland. Jews from Bessarabia, Romania, immigrated their from Poland and the Ukraine in the 18th century. Sephardic Jews from Constantinople had already immigrated to Romania around 1506.

There were distant ancestors in Transylvania, Poland, Moldova. I emerged myself in books and music, in art and writing. Creative expression is all that there is, and where love is to be found.

Would knowing the history of the Portuguese Marrano Society of London be of use later? And later I dreamed at twelve that when I grew up I wrote about the secret Marrano brand of Judaism found in Portuguese village life today. I wrote about Jews in Egypt and dressed in the customary fashion, and my Zamba Mora dances, my Indic dances, my Biblical dances, like my music, healed the mind and body. Why should it make such a difference? But to the clique it did.

West First Street in Brooklyn forked into the right side of the street lined with four-family apartment houses of poor Polish Jews, across the subway tracks near Kings Highway. On the left side resided block after block of Italian Catholics, mostly from Naples or Sicily and a few Greeks and Armenians about a mile away.

Later, I had my mtDNA tested, and found it matched with the Italians from Siena in Tuscany and Greeks from Crete. The Syrians with whom I went to junior high school would live in private houses by choice about ten blocks away. They owned their electronic and clothing businesses. They didn't work as janitors in coal bins mopping toilets in the Navy Yard at midnight like my father did. I had to have something to hold my head up for.

The Polish Jews wouldn't have my family. I started to read about the Spanish and Portuguese secret Jews and their secret prayers held over for five hundred years. I read about the villages of Braganca, Oporto, Rebordello, Belmonte. Secret Jews in secret Sabbath. But where does a Polish Jewish girl fit into a Syrian Jewish women's class on reading the portion of Torah?

I never told anyone in class that my grandparents were Polish Jews from Lodz and Bialystok. I was a Bialystoker, but I admired the Syrian Jews in my class for their exhilarating dance music records, their delicious foods, and the spices. I made my own Lebanese spices with allspice, black pepper, cinnamon, nutmeg, cardamom, cloves, ginger, and dried rose petals and mixed it ground in a spice grinder, on most of my food. I liked it better than Polish Jewish Babka cake, kasha knishes from Brighton Beach, stuffed kishke, gefilte fish, and roast chicken with carrot 'tsimma.'

But Aleppo's! These Syrian Jews had mansions and money and ceremony. "Why can't I join your sorority? The Meegahs looks like lots of fun!"

"You gotta be Syrian to join," Busta smirked.

"Well what if I said I was Syrian?"

"You gotta be from Aleppo. We don't even let the Damascus Jews join because some of their people were dancing girls."

"Bullshine." I cracked my knuckles in Busta's face. Busta, the balabusta, (the thorough housewife) the Polish Jews in my class called her.

"You ain't got any Syrian name."

"That doesn't mean anything. What if I had a stepfather or something'? What about some of you with your Italian and Spanish names? Not all of you have Arab names."

"I haven't seen you around any Syrian neighborhoods. You don't live near our neighborhood or on any of the surrounding streets."

"Don't you people ever read about your own history? I spend days in the library reading all about you people."

"You don't even go to the Syrian synagogue." Busta rolled her gold-flecked brown eyes at Seeley and nudged elbows with her friend. I took it as a put-down."

"How do you know what synagogue I go to?"

"Your family doesn't go to our Nobeh parties. And you wear lipstick. I've never seen you around before."

"What would I have to do to join your sorority? I stared over Seeley's shoulder, unable to look into her playpen eyes.

"Pass initiation. You have to take off all your clothes in Seeley's closet and let her six-year old brother feel you up."

"I couldn't do such a thing."

"Did you ever let a boy feel you up?" Busta giggled and bit off the eraser of her pencil. Seeley giggled so hard she began to sneeze.

"Is that your stupid initiation rites?"

"You have to take off your sweater and bra in Seeley' closet and walk into her living room and stand there while Waynie feels you up."

"And fingerprints you." Seeley giggled.

"What about your mother?"

Seeley cringed. "She's in Florida for a week. The cleaning lady finishes the ironing at two and leaves for three hours to go shopping."

My face went rubbery. Seeley began to pull out loose eyelashes. If I take off my clothes, are you sure I can join the Meegahs?"

"Do you want to join?" Busta whispered as the home room break period was ending.

"You're pretty weird."

To be a Syrian Jewish Princess was all that mattered. I kept it hidden, the desire to be a Jewish princess. Here I was the queen of the Gypsies to my inner self, living on La Caminita de la reyna de los Gitanos, living on the street of the Queen of the Gypsies in my inner dollhouse. No one else around was rich like that. Rich in Brazil. Rich in Brooklyn.

Daddy's darling rich. Being Syrian meant you had a caring daddy, a generous daddy who shelled out the money for Nobeh parties. Your mother had married a generous and kind man, slow to anger. Oh, if only I had a daddy whose temper wouldn't go from zero to ten in an instant, if only mom and I didn't have to walk on egg shells to stay alive.

The leaders of the Meegahs: Seeley,-Robrana, Wiley, and Busta, met at Seeley's house on the main strip of the Syrian neighborhood. Everyone I knew at thirteen went to the same junior high eighth-grade class. But no parents were present in the large mansion. The smiling black maid in a white uniform finished ironing the last of the laundry and left to do her round of shopping.

Each of the young ladies settled down on the velvety, white sofa with the black pillows while Seeley served the Syrian Pizzas-a heated pocket of pita bread dripping with spiced feta cheese, olive oil, and roasted sweet red peppers, onions, mushrooms, and fried pine (pignola) nuts.

I heard all of your parents come from just one city in Syria-Aleppo." I paced the floor nervously, looking around the mansion.

Seeley nodded and glanced, wide-eyed at Busta. I caught Busta's cold stare and pondered her turtle-bean-black eyes.

Several times Seeley and Busta exchanged silent glances and nudged each other's elbows, giggling by habit. I spoke nervously in front of the overflowing Syrian synagogue on Yom Kippur. "How's it going, folks?" I had wanted them to be family so eagerly, I called them folks and then felt out of sync for doing so.

"It's an esnoga. We don't call it a synagogue or a schule like the Polish Jews. If you were Syrian you'd know it was called la esnoga." Seeley's voice was a soft, seductive, compelling beat.

"Esnoga?" I laughed loudly. "What if I told you my parents are directly from Spain to Salonika? We still speak Ladino, old Spanish, not Arabic. And you're telling me it's an esnoga?" Yet I knew my father came from Bialystock, spoke Yiddish, and my mother, tired of being beaten by my dad, decided to try out the Christian religion and dragged me to all the churches.

"When the holocaust comes back to Brooklyn to burn the children black," mom always said, "If they find out you're Jewish, it will be a true test of human nature what they will do with you. Better change your name and tell the world you're Welsh. You look Welsh."

"But I look more like I come from northern India than from Wales," I said.

We ended up in the Unitarian church. I remembered from the age of three that mom would hold me and warn, "The bombs will come to New York. Someday a power will come here and get you for looking Jewish. I have to decorate the house in Shamrocks and tell everyone I'm Irish."

"The real Jews come from Syria," Seeley continued proudly. "We've been there for more than two thousand years." Polish Jews are self-styled and come from the West Slavic Sorbs of Lusatia in Eastern Germany, near the Polish border. It's in a lot of history books. Charlemagne's son tried to turn the Sorbs Christian, and some of them joined the Jews in German villages during the ninth century. It's in the books. They turned Jewish rather late, not four thousand years ago, like us Syrians. We're real. Why do you think there are so many blue-eyed redheads and blondes among North Eastern European Jews?"

"I see in this class three blue-eyed blondes among Syrian Jews," I answered.

"But we're real Jews." Seeley showed me a history book. "Like the Jews of Iraq."

"And I'm not real?" My voice was cracking.

"You're a European Jew."

"What if I say I'm as Jewish as you are?"

"No, you have North Central European blood."

"How can you know what blood I have? You're just thirteen."

"I look more Biblical Jewish than you do. I bet you have German blood. I heard that people who have German blood turn gray much earlier than those who have Middle Eastern blood."

Busta handed me a piece of Syrian pizza. "We're all Syrian. Our sorority is only for Syrian girls-Jewish, orthodox, people that live here, people we know, people who don't use lipstick in the eighth grade."

I twisted in the chair. "Have you ever been to the Syrian social center?"

"We're building another Syrian social center for this neighborhood." Busta tossed a glob of melted cheese in her mouth.

"I hear Avy Joseph is practicing for his Bar Mitzvah right now." Just a few doors away stood the holiest synagogue.

"You know what you have to do right now. Initiation time." Seeley cracked her gum.

"Sure. Where's your closet?"

It was dark in the hallway as I snuggled into Seeley's huge closet packed with fragrance and the most expensive Bloomingdale's clothes. She peeled off her red sweater and torn undershirt.

"What are you doing in there so long?" Seeley shouted, a bit frightened that I was marking or sticking gum on her clothes or worse.

"I'm ready."

After an eternity of torment, I walked out nude from the waist up, clutching my mangled undershirt and faded sweater to my concave, underdeveloped chest. At last I revealed that I was flat-chested/small breasted forever and wore a padded bra to fill out my clothes. Imagine what that feels like at thirteen in the eighth grade in front of a large group of girls you have to see every day in our middle school class.

Busta pulled my sweater and shirt out of my grip as I watched myself in the mirror, a frail, five-foot girl crossing her arms over her chest to hide her flat breasts, pallor, and obvious lack of estrogen.

Poor nutrition had created narrow bones, and I was at least two years behind in development. My pitiful sight made the other girls want to peck and dominate the runt of the litter. Only the pubescent had the popularity. On top of it, how could I let them know who I really am? That nobody taught me morals, only to stay away from boys. I stayed away and read the books. I also had never had a friend.

Busta tossed her clothing high in the air to Seeley, then to Robrana and to Wiley. The sweater and undershirt went back and forth between the interknot of girls as they blocked the doorway so that there was nowhere I could escape.

"Volley ball. Volley ball," Seeley shouted.

"Monkey in the middle. Monkey in the middle," Busta sang mockingly.

"Give me back my clothes. Please, girls," I gasped, running back and forth between Seeley and Busta as they tossed my clothing over my head. The girls towered over me. Wiley and Robrana stood on the side and watched, waving their arms, blocking my path.

I tried to get some eye contact with any of the girls, to find some connection, just a trace of humanity. But they wouldn't permit it. There was no way I could extract any caring from them, not for me, anyway.

I flitted from girl to girl, but they locked me outside their playpen eyes. They stared at a point over my shoulder and waved their hands over my head.

"Where's your six-year-old brother? You lied to me. He's not here. He'd tell your parents on you," I screamed.

Wiley gave a Bronx cheer. "Her sweater-go on, give it to her," one girl shouted.

"Hey Busta. Give her back her sweater." Beady-eyed Busta flung the sweater at my feet. Then she held up the wash-worn undershirt and peered through the hole it had ... "Yuk! It stinks," Busta pretended, taking a long whiff of the cotton. She tossed it up in the air.

I reached up to catch the sweater and shirt in mid-air. The girls giggled loudly.

"Look how small her breasts are. Flat as a pancake." Seeley made a groan of disgust. The rest of the girls stopped in their tracks to stare at my concave chest and convex belly, just like my father had, as I struggled to pull on my child-like undershirt and then the loose sweater.

"Aren't you old enough to use a deodorant?" Seeley laughed.

"Sure, rubbing alcohol and baking soda all the time."

In spite of the ridicule, I only sensed the undercurrent that pulled me toward the family-like clique I envied. It was the mouth-watering smell of the good Columbian coffee percolating and the heat waves of the chocolate chip cookies in the oven that Seeley was baking for the sorority before discussion time.

I had never smelled those home-baking smells at my house. Our own oven broke in 1946 and stood that way. We ate instant coffee or cocoa, or cookies stale in their wrappers from the thrift market, no homemade food that had lingering smells other than frying eggs in melted white fat or boiled chicken that tasted like cardboard.

Busta brought my senses back to reality. "We have no initiation rites to join the,Meegahs. We just wanted to see how crazy you'd act to get into our sorority."

It wasn't at all like I had imagined. "You really went and did it."

"Why did you lie and keep insisting you were Syrian? I know where you live," Seeley sneered, "in a roach-wracked apartment next to the subway ... and not in the Syrian neighborhood."

I stepped back toward the door, too embarrassed to think. "I'll have to face you in school tomorrow and for the rest of the year."

Busta spit her gum in a tissue, laughing. "Crazy is really nuts enough to get naked to join our club."

"Crazy," Wiley laughed.

"You mean you don't like me, even a little, not even like a sister?" I whined softly like a mouse.

Busta opened the door and shoved me into the street. I backed up and the four girls paced toward until I stood at the curb. Then Busta tossed her into the street into the path of an oncoming car. The car braked and came to a halt only a few inches before hitting me, but it missed. A guardian angel on my shoulder protected me. It never left me, and I felt its presence always after that.

The next thing I looked up only to see Avy Joseph, the Syrian Jewish boy who's father owned the biggest business I ever heard of, coming out of the Syrian synagogue where he'd been practicing for his Bar Mitzvah.

I had a crush on Avy for a year. I walked over to get a closer look at his tan face and big, black cow eyes, the thick golden chestnut hair, and his tall, athletic body. Avy wore his prayer shawl and skullcap, too holy to talk to at the moment.

The girls walked down the block, giggling, and I was left standing alone to face Avy walking toward me.

"Hello Avy, how is school?" I couldn't stop myself from talking to him. The car that braked to a stop now became attached to a man who kept tooting his horn and screaming … "You crazy schlemiel. Want to get killed? Goddamn kids. Idiot." But I ran away from the clamor and toward angel-faced Avy.

"Wouldn't you even give me the time of day?" Avy didn't even look up at me. "How is your Bar Mitzvah rehearsal going?"

"Pretty good," he said quickly and softly, hurrying on his way to the crowd of girls waiting for him at the corner. His prayer shawl shivered in the breeze, the fringes dancing back and forth as he walked from the hips.

At the end of the block I watched him from a distance as he crossed his ankles and leaned against the stone fence of his house with a girl on each side. I passed them all, smiling and chatting like what they had to say was the most important thing in their world and it was. Nobody looked my way. I couldn't think of anything but the dimples in Avy's smooth cheeks when he smiled at someone else.

4

MY PARENT'S APARTMENT, 1955

By the time I got home, mother had begun to sort out the way-too-small nighties and rhinestone earrings she had shoplifted from some downtown Brooklyn Heights department store. I stormed in, still shaking from the ordeal with Seeley and the eighth-grade junior high sorority.

"I'm damn tired of your shoplifting, mom!" I let it all out on mother, looking askance at the dangling earrings Tsipke was holding against her ear lobe, gazing in the foyer mirror.

Tsipke raked her daughter with her large, silver eyes with the tiny flecks of dark brown. "Benjamin passed the bar. So now he's a lawyer," she announced. "That means you'll have to be quiet when he works in the foyer."

"In this tiny two-bedroom apartment? Can't he study anymore in the storage room down in the cellar?"

"No. It's bad for his asthma."

I put my astronomy and anthropology books about Neanderthal life from the library away in the bedroom I now shared with my 26-year old brother.

"So he's getting married soon. What nerve. Instead of getting a furnished room for his bride, he's bringing her here until they finish building his house. Now I get thrown out and have to sleep on the stinky sofa where the dog pissed."

Tsipke looked over her shoulder at me. "It won't be for more than a couple of months."

"Sure." I sighed. "I hate that bitch he's going to marry-hate her for throwing me out of my room. What kind of a man brings his bride here?"

Tsipke looked in the mirror again with a cigarette dangling from her vivid red lips. "She's inviting you to her wedding, isn't she? Making you second maid of honor."

Tsipke put some beads around her neck and then took them off and hung them around the white column of my throat.

"Get those cheap, wax beads out of here. And that sugary perfume is sickening. I told you they got the evil eye. They're cursed, mom, cursed. You'll get bad luck."

"How else can I live on the three dollars a day your father leaves on the refrigerator?"

"You know what you look like stuffing nighties into your pants?"

Tsipke scratched the corners of her parted lips and looked at me through half-closed lids. "You think I wanted you? Damn. You were born just as I was about to divorce your father. I'm taking care of you just because it's my responsibility."

"You hate kids, don't you?" I sneered.

"So do you."

"Don't worry. I won't have any. I won't get married. I hate men. And I feel real mean to older women also."

"You're just like your old man."

"I'm scared of children, scared I'11 catch chicken pox from them as an old lady and blow away."

"I was just about to get a job in the winding factory-winding thread on giant spools-just like when I was a young girl. Then at thirty-eight I found out I was pregnant, with you."

I went into the kitchen and Tsipke followed me, taunting. "Horseface"

I turned to mother. "What do you get from shoplifting? Some kind of sexual excitement?" I grabbed the broom and swung it in circles.

"You know a lot for thirteen."

"Really? Then why do you keep complaining to me, nagging me like I was a man-that you haven't had any since I was born? Why do you think I have to know that?"

"Because your father never has taken a bath." The two women stood silent for a moment. Then Tsipke slapped me across the face as she always did when I pushed all her wrong buttons.

"Sometimes I wonder how I was ever conceived." I didn't bother to cry anymore in front of her mother.

"My father paid us a visit."

Mother and daughter finally sat down opposite each other in the kitchen. "What has that got to do with it?"

"I was so happy to see him after so many years. He left my step mother when I was ten and disappeared. My real mother gave me away when I was two."

Tsipke's face beamed and she drifted off into another world. "My own parents were divorced when I was two. Mom gave me away to my father and he took me to Philadelphia. He disappeared for so many years." He spent so little time with me, dumping me on the woman he lived with. I ate out of garbage cans."

I was beginning to understand these mother-daughter chats. "So you were so glad to see your father that you allowed your husband to make love to you that night and I was conceived."

Tsipke looked up for a moment. "It would be different if I were married to a caring man."

"And what about this scar?" I turned my chin towards Tsipke.

"What about the scar you made on my face when I said you were as ugly as your old man?"

"You shouldn't have cut me down like that," I whined.

"Mouse, you had no right to throw your math compass or was it a protractor-in your mother's face."

"Well I failed math three times already, doesn't that even out your curse?"

"You shouldn't have disobeyed me."

"And that's why I fell over that schoolyard fence and split my chin open." I began to eat the snacks on the table.

"You fell over the fence because you were playing some fantasy game with a Syrian girl. I told you time and time again that Syrians are bad luck for you. She was with you when you ran and fell. You must have done something pretty bad to Syrians in a previous life to be punished so every time you try to be friends with one."

I stared for a long while at mother and began to talk about that advice. "It wasn't my curse. I wasn't anywhere near there."

"I was bad the day before. I can't remember what I said to you, because I was only nine. I did something and you put a curse on me for it."

"No. It was the Syrians, from some former life. An ancient curse. You did something to them and that's why they're bringing you bad luck now."

I walked about the kitchen. "The Syrian girl simply said 'let's pretend the janitor is chasing us. Let's run and climb over fences and pretend and hide. We were two nine-year olds playing pretend. I was only in the fourth grade, mom. Would curses stretch so far to children?"

Tsipke let out a guffaw. "The little Syrian bitch made you climb a fence that swung open and you lost your balance and split your face open. Can't you see the curse? She wanted to fire up her fantasy at your expense."

"Will Syrians always bring me bad luck? Then why do I want to marry, one-like Avy Joseph-so much? At the same time I'm warned by some inner feeling that I should never marry, never have children, and never ride on a-plane. My fear is so great to do these things, mom. Is there an angel that's warning me not to marry or have children or ride in an airplane? I felt so strongly about this since I was seven. I even wrote it down on a pad and locked it in the nightstand to remind me when I grow up."

"Stop already." Tsipke yelled. "We shouldn't even bring back her name. She's a jinx.

"What did dad mean when he told you he should have flushed me out into the bay before I was born?"

"He meant if I only had used birth control, you wouldn't be here. And I'd swing free." I turned on the radio to classical music.

"My father loved the opera. He was a classical music conductor, you know-in the old country," said Tsipke.

"Free to do what-make lopsided ashtrays, mom?"

"Such complications from you! Why do I have to be dragged into these talks?" Tsipke began to run water for her coffee pot.

"The day I married, I wrote in my diary: "today I died.' Your old man found my diary on our honeymoon train to Florida. He gave me my diary back with tears in his eyes. If I died the day I got married, then were you born from my ashes?"

"Mom. Tell me. Why are you afraid to be Jewish? Or Jewish? it's okay in this country, you know. They're not going to get you."

"Shut up!" Tsipke screeched. "Do you know how many times your grandmother had her ears boxed in America for just looking Jewish? What if they found out she had been Jewish before that? Beaten by total strangers! And as they were kicking her, she was screaming, 'But I'm Portuguese, I'm Portuguese!' Maybe she should have said Armenian instead or Greek or Italian. Maybe even Georgian. Why do so many people from Northern Europe pull back oddly when close to someone from Southern Europe?

"Is the war between the Paleolithic hunters of Ice Age Europe still raging at the Neolithic farmers for moving into their territory from Anatolia or Central Asia?" I questioned mom, "And me? They said I had the map of Jerusalem printed on my Jewish face," she continued, ignoring my reference to my anthropology hobby. "Could it have been my curly black hair or my grey eyes with those dark brown flecks in them?" She looked at her face in the mirror, running her hand over her mouth to silence herself. "If I didn't have a stepmother ... and didn't have to eat out of garbage cans and catch diphtheria ..."

"Boy," I wheezed. So what if your step mother reared you? She came from Odessa, and that redhead is Jewish, and so is your father from Lodz, in Poland, and he wanted to be a doctor, I heard. Daddy's from Bialystok. Yet your dad became a classical and opera orchestra conductor." How come he ended up owning a fruit stand? I wonder what it must have been like in the old country for grandma."

"This doesn't only happen in a Jewish family," Tsipke said." What did you do about grandma?"

"I waited twenty-eight years later until you were born and then I put on a cross. Grandma used to sell cloth to the nuns. But it wasn't nuns who bothered her. It was the school kids she saw every day and their parents.

"The fear of being hurt never stops," Tsipke sighed. "You won't get out of your own way. Daddy still beats you in the home."

7

Dance Hall at the YMCA New York City, August 1963

Saturn was in Aquarius in my fifth house of romance and creativity, and the dance floor was not crowded that Saturday night at the foreign student's dance. The Irish Jew who was getting his PhD in Spanish put on an African dance and drums record and I, now twenty one, began to row my elbows back and forth as I danced alone to the Angolan rhythms.

I grew up to be a five-foot-four, slender woman with hip-length reddish black curls, porcelain complexion, and dove-like hazel eyes set in the ancient Mediterranean face of a Spanish grandee, a Gypsy face with freckled, pale yellow skin.

Couples watched as I danced alone in African style, my silk Chinese beads bobbing across a royal blue satin blouse. Then someone removed the Olatunji record and put on the twist.

Malek was a green-eyed, chestnut-haired exchange student from Lebanon. I had met him a few times before at these international student dances where I hunted the foreign talent for a fresh outlook on simple conversation. How did the other half live and what did it feel like? These were the questions I probed the tourists and foreign students for, and they were only too happy to respond. At international student dances in New York City, you'll find all ethnic types and immigrants.

This was 1963, and Malek said he was a Druze from Lebanon. He introduced me to his friend, a Muslim from Syria in New York only six weeks, a man who was to become my first husband. He assumed I was an Arab American just by looking at me. I had to tell him my parents are Jewish from Poland. Honesty is the best policy. The man he introduced me to appeared not to care. I wondered how desperate was he to stay in America, that a Syrian Arab Muslim would ask a Jewish American girl from a Hasidic family from Bialystok, a girl who loved going to the Lubavitcher Chabad synagogue, to marry him? He said he wasn't religious and my religion wouldn't matter.

Why was I drawn to keep dating him, to believe him? I knew him only six weeks and then married him? Why did I do that at twenty-one when I had not really dated before? Was I that desperate to get away from parents who were frequently fighting? I didn't realize my dad was suffering from "elder rage" and taking it out on my mom.

I had won a scholarship to an Ivy League college, made membership into Mensa, the high IQ society, and was finishing my junior year as a visual anthropology/archaeology and professional writing double major and a film school minor with a second minor in personality psychology and illustration. I loved studying the Renaissance and humanities and lived for the coming-of age of women in film, as executives behind the scenes while reading Friedan's "The Feminine Mystique."

This summer I tutored Malek in technical documentary film writing and play directing, two courses in which he was not sure of his footing in English. Malek was twenty-eight and we had dated platonically for weeks. It was 1963, before the feminists were described as "bitter" by the doctor's daughters in my creative writing class who showed me their engagement rings. Almost everyone in my college class was either Jewish or Italian. My closest friend was a shy Greek girl. I used to go with another Greek gal pal to Greek school when I was nine or ten. We had a lot in common, like making rolled grape leaves. Deja vue. In a former life, I felt, I'd done this before in Athens.

Back at the International Student dance, Malek saw me undulating to the sob shocks of a Congo drum and quickly approached. "Thanks again for the help," Malek teased. He was more interested in the buxom blonde with whom I had traveled to the dance. "How about introducing me to your friend?"

Andrea, at twenty-three was the daughter of a holocaust survivor, a Polish Jew. She only dated Jewish doctors, mostly those just coming from Iran who might tend to marry a Jewish girl without money.

So I introduced Andrea to Malek. But when he asked the Marilyn Monroe look-alike to dance, she told him she was waiting for this Iranian Jewish medical doctor who played Klezmer violin to relax who was supposed to meet her there.

"Are you German?" Malek asked Andrea. "No. I'm a Polish Jew." With that Malek was taken aback by Andrea's forthright statement.

I explained, "Malek, Andrea only dates foreign Jewish doctors from exotic countries like Samarkand or Iran or Turkey."

"Because the ones born here want wives whose fathers are wealthy enough to set them up in business or training," I added.

"Oh, I see. It would be easier to marry an Arab doctor who wants to come here," Malek laughed.

"Doctor?" my ears perked up.

"She's joking," Andrea blurted.

Galosh got himself a soft drink. "Say, I have a friend I'd like you to meet. He just came from Syria only five days ago. He's a doctor-of mechanical engineering. Name's Ahmed Haddad* (name is changed for privacy), a Muslim."

I looked sideways at Malek's friend. "Sure, I'll meet him."

"Doesn't speak a word of English, though." Malek added.

"You're kidding!" I swished my skirt with impatience. "The only word in Arabic I know is Habibi."

Malek looked disturbed. "I'll interpret. Besides he wants to learn English. Will you help him?" I agreed.

"Say, how come you stopped dating me?" Malek looked at her askance.

"You dropped out of college. You're an airplane mechanic. I told you I'm looking to marry a professional man who'll be a good provider." I smiled. "I want somebody stable who won't drag me down to their factory job level."

"Too bad. But what makes you think a professional man would want you?"

"After I worked so hard in the library to put myself through college at night, Don't I deserve a good provider with interesting conversation?"

Andrea broke up the argument. "Hey, we all go into marriage looking for a package deal."

"So is that going to make you rich?" Malek frowned. "You make me feel castrated. Anyhow, Here he is."

Malek spoke in Arabic to Ahmed Haddad who waited on the sidelines. The three-way conversation was conducted through Galosh.

"So you're really a doctor of engineering?" I chuckled. Talking through Malek, Ahmed look at me and beamed. "I'm only here five days from Syria." He had smiling green eyes and curly chocolate brown hair, a peach complexion and stocky build.

"He's twenty-six," Malek added.

Ahmed's eyes seemed to never stop laughing. His stapled smile never quivered.

"What do you see we all go to the all-night automat to talk?" Malek suggested.

The last thing I wanted was to go home on a Saturday night to the bleak apartment where my father waited to scream at me that I used too much toilet paper or I ate too much food. "You're eating me out of house and home," he would cliché a thousand times a year. For a second his words fleshed out in my mind. "You must have a mighty big hole there to have to use so much toilet paper," he'd shout. Meyer never stopped calling me a tramp.

And my mother was-in Florida for the winter recuperating from her hardening arteries. I remained a virgin until my wedding night, and nobody gave a damn that I waited and enjoyed staying a good little girl and would for a lifetime if I could only find a secure job that could become like a family. No, I didn't look forward to going back to her apartment on this humid night.

Meyer was becoming more violent. After a series of strokes his brain tissue damage was increasing to the point where I feared living at home much longer.

At least mother had got out for the several months. For sixty-five dollars a month, she had rented a room in Miami alone and for the first time in her life wasn't battered or belittled every day. She could finally be the Jewish girl her grandmother was, if only it would lead to the path of comfort and nourishment.

Malek, Ahmed Haddad, and I bolted with exuberance as we leaped on the subway and rode toward the Times Square automat.

We sat and talked and laughed. Before I knew it, the last bus back to Hoboken, New Jersey was leaving at three in the morning. And Malek had to make that bus. Ahmed was staying with him. He didn't know what else to do but to put me on the subway, alone, at Times Square.

The two men left me at the subway turnstile and paid my fare home with a subway token. I was miffed. Isn't anyone going to put me in a taxi or take me home like a gentleman?"

I couldn't believe two men would drop a young lady off in Times Square at three in the morning for a ride alone back to Coney Island on the D Train.

Suddenly I realized that someone snatched the money I always tuck into my purse when I go out—to get home alone safely by cab—from Manhattan to Brooklyn. Maybe the purse opened and the money fell out by itself. Without judging, I begged Malek to take me home or at least lend me money for cab fare until the next day. He insisted that he make the last bus home to Hoboken so he wouldn't have to be out alone himself all night and also in danger in the New York City streets.

Ahmed didn't speak much English and could have been from anywhere. He went along with Malek since he was in New York alone, didn't know too many people, and only in the US only a few days. I understood. Two guys from the Middle East meet an American Jewish girl. They talk. They go home. Neither wanted to be on the streets of New York at three in the morning, and none had taken enough money for a cab, only with bus fare and a desire to grab that last bus back to Hoboken, New Jersey.

I had a subway token of my own and fifteen cents in change, not enough for a cab. Nobody could be called. I went into the subway and caught the D Train toward Coney Island.

In my spike heels and white satin and lace fancy suit, I made her way into the subway car and sat opposite a middle-aged black man wearing a working man's cap. All I noticed was the scar on his cheek.

I didn't notice the two or three other men on the train, since I had hid my face against the window, turning from the man's view to avoid eye contact and trouble. He probably thought I deserved to get what he would dish out because I dared to be a woman of 21 who tried to take back the night. I dared to be riding the subway at three AM on a cold, February, snowy morning.

Why did I ever stay so late dancing and talking? Why didn't the guys take me home? I thought about it. An American guy would have brought me home, any guy would if he had planned a date. This wasn't a date. I met two men, chatted, and each went our own way to get home. How dare I assume they would take me home just because I sat and talked with them or danced until three in the morning?

The man sitting across from me in the subway stepped off at King's Highway, a few stops before Coney Island, when I exited at that station to go home. As I stepped off the subway, peering around, I didn't see anything. But out of a corner of my eye, I thought I saw him dart behind the huge bench signs. I was too tired to pay attention.

I waited a few minutes in the station near the turnstile. There was a night attendant there who made change. Nobody followed me down. After a long while, I walked down the metal stairs to Kings Highway and walked the two blocks to my apartment on West First Street past the candy store and the Kosher butcher.

Suddenly the black man sneaked up behind me unheard and unseen. Right in front of the vacant, weed-filled lot he put his hand on my shoulder.

"Hi baby," the man sneered with a sardonic smile.

I twisted my neck and stared at him, then bolted in her spike heels across the lot toward her home. Right in front of my apartment he caught up with me, dragged me back into the weeds of the lot and began to strangle me. I pretended to go limp and close my eyes and his grip loosened a bit. Then he pulled off my glasses and stomped them into bits.

"Here, take my money," I gasped. "He grabbed the bag and tossed it over his shoulder. Four cents jingled in my purse. That's all the money I had. Then he dragged me to the curb so I'd be hidden by a parked car.

I started to give a little scream, but he yelled "Shut up you bitch!" and started to strangle me again.

He loosened his grip as soon as I would feign going limp and closing her eyes. He laid me down alongside the curb and looked into her eyes what seemed like a long while as he put his finger into the side of her panties and then into my vagina.

There was an obstacle. At twenty-one, I was a virgin and remained so until my wedding. He couldn't go far with his finger, because he found out soon enough that I had an intact hymen. So after watching the frown on my face for a moment, he started to choke me again. Before I could react and pretend to go limp to make him loosen his grip, somehow the window above the parked car opened with a loud screech.

The man jumped up and bolted away into the night, dropping his workman's cap. All that was left was my purse that he dropped and the fragments of my crushed eyeglasses in the lot.

"Call the police," I called to my neighbor, the old Polish Jewish woman who opened the window. "Good Mrs. Kutkowski." A woman in her eighties who spoke with a thick, Yiddish accent spoke to me as the man ran away, dropping his hat.

The neighbor called the police for me. "Did you hear me start to scream?" I wanted to know.

But Mrs. Kutkowksi shook her head "not' and just opened the window for some air because she couldn't sleep. What made her open the window to get some air at that instant, saving my life?

"Are you all right?" she said in her sing-song inclination. "I wish all you pishi-kas (teenage girls) wouldn't sit out on the stoop and fool around all night.'

"I said I was nearly strangled!" I fumed. "And I'm not going back into my apartment until I've seen a doctor."

"What about your father?" She insisted.

"I don't want to be in there with him." I called back to her from the street. "He has this elder rage problem. Loses his temper and explodes at people for no reason and chases them with a hammer."

I waited what seemed like an eternity for the police to arrive. When the first officer arrived he asked I to explain.

"Were you raped?"

"No. He tried to strangle me." I told him about his fingers in my vagina. "Could I get VD?" I asked.

"Look, if your boyfriend got fresh with you and you want to get revenge, don't send us on a wild goose chase."

I was incredulous. Why wouldn't the police officer believe my word straight on? February 1963 was the year, not 1862. It was the first time I had ever spoken with a policeman. What reason could I have for making this up? I thought.

"My boyfriend?" I looked at the officer as if I had learned that I could never trust another man again, another relationship, another date. "If I had a boyfriend to protect me, this wouldn't ever have happened."

"I just wanted to be sure," the police answered defensively.

The second officer searched about the weedy lot and found her crushed glasses and the man's cap. He brought it over for the first officer to examine. "Looks like the kind of caps they wear."

The first officer then began to take me a little more seriously. He asked me who I was, age and occupation. "I'm a visual anthropology and English-writing emphasis-graphic design triple major," I told him. "I want to be a creative director."

They left. There was nothing more they could do. The man had run away towards the subway station and the trains had come and gone many times before the police car arrived. "You must have quite an imagination," the officer said curtly. "I sure hope your boyfriend didn't do this and you're out for revenge."

"I told you if I had a boyfriend to protect me, this wouldn't have happened." I still wanted to see men as the protector. Only the reality is all the men in my life made me feel unsafe and frightened both in the home and in the outside world. What was left? The imagined safety and security of the job.

Yes, in 1963, jobs in New York were still as easy to find as they were in the fifties when I was in high school. I had a job in the library checking out magazines. It was safe and quiet in the middle of Times Square. I did my job, earned my tuition to supplement the scholarship, but it didn't pay enough for me to have my own apartment. I still lived at home with my parents, and that was wearing thin.

I went back to my parent's apartment and sneaked in. Dad slept soundly. And in my bed after a silent and quick wash-up, the black and blue thumb prints on my neck where I'd been choked began to throb. He damaged my thyroid, I thought. Anxiety overtook me, and the life-long lasting panic disorder and over-stimulated thyroid, my big oversized thyroid, began its journey to panic land and chronic anxiety. I gasped for breath each time I had tried to lean back on the pillow in the dark listening to the blood coursing through my arteries. If only I found a diet to soothe my nerves. To be alone was glorious. Solitude meant safety and serenity. Music therapy said it all with calmness. Finally I phoned for a police ambulance. After an eternity, it arrived. This time I dressed and waited downstairs, so Meyer wouldn't wake up with a commotion.

"My neck feels like it's damaged," I told the ambulance driver before he even got out of the driver's seat.

"Are you the one?" The driver opened the door for her.

"I have a sociology exam on Monday. And now this. Say, can I catch VD from his hand? Am I still a virgin?" These questions went through my mind as the ambulance drove toward Coney Island hospital. Happy twenty-first birthday to me.

There was a light exam at the hospital. "Not unless he scratched you," was the nurse's answer to her VD question. "After all, the only thing that went inside was his fingers."

"It's my neck I'm worried about. I can't swallow properly." The blue thumb-prints on my throat began to swell.

"I don't want my father to find out. He'll get violent." I told the doctor, "He'll call me a whore."

"You'll be okay," the hospital attendant assured me as I left the emergency room. There was no counseling, no mention of rape or even sexual assault. Nothing spoken. "There's no damage," she was assured.

"What about my neck? It's all bruised."

"I said you're o.k." The emergency room nurse began to lose her patience.

"No I'm not," I squealed. "You're going to send me a bill for fifty bucks for the ambulance ride, plus the cost of the emergency room exam. I won't be able to face my job in the library Monday morning. I'll probably get a "D" on my sociology exam. How come I get attacked and it costs me money?"

"You're lucky you weren't murdered," the answer came back.

"Lucky?" I walked down the long corridors to a waiting taxi I called-totally flattened and desperately looking for a protector to marry as quickly as I could find him, any him. Come Monday, I received a "B-plus" in sociology, then called Ahmed and brought up the subject of marriage. Somebody had better take care of me fast, I fantasized in paralogic.

8

Darlene's House, September 1963

Darlene was a famous judge's single, twenty-five year old daughter who lived in the plushest, private house with a black maid in the suburbs of New York. They called it Jamaica Estates, and the house was bought for seventy-five thousand dollars many years before 1963.

The first thing I noticed about my friend's house was that she said her parents paid seventy-five thousand dollars for the house years ago. The house looked enormous to me, decorated with Darlene's interior designing mom's paintings.

For a moment I imagined myself as an accomplished interior designed married to a rich lawyer or doctor or judge like Darlene's mom. Only Darlene had emotional problems and saw a therapist because she could afford a therapist. Her parents paid her bills. At twenty-five, she didn't work for pay and took courses now and then in sociology at the university I went to.

Darlene was my best friend in college before Darlene dropped out of her sociology major to travel and husband-hunt in the Catskills. She had lost interest in her fashion design classes, dropped out of her bilingual secretarial school, and finally, dropped out of the sociology department at New York University and got a job as a clerk typist in Greenwich Village.

Like me, Darlene was Jewish from Eastern European grandparents. Only Darlene said she was secular and dated Lebanese and Turkish Muslim men as well as Jewish men, most of whom she met in the Catskill resorts. The Muslim men she met at various university functions. In high-school she dated a Lebanese Christian man. His parents wouldn't let him marry her, but she told me she loved him.

Now she was dating Jewish men she met at Grossinger's in the Catskills. I have never been to the Catskills. It costs money, and I had only enough for college tuition, clothes, food, subway fare, and books. I'd never had a vacation that lasted more than one or two days, and the only place I'd been was to Asbury Park, Atlantic City, or Washington, DC for sightseeing or a different beach.

I never dropped out of any school. Just the thought of not graduating from a university made me shiver. I'd end up like mom who dropped out of the fifth grade, seeking jobs in beauty parlors as a maid or not working at all, pretending to be a lady instead of a woman. A lady had a husband to support her.

A woman had to work because her husband was too weak to take care of her was what mom told me. I wanted to be a lady, but I didn't dare to imagine finding a man to support me. I looked too much like Woody Allen for a man to get interested in my flat chest/small breasts, large, convex nose, scarred face, and poverty. For a man to get interested in me, I needed money or a trust fund or rich parents. In college, at least I was working toward a community college teaching credential.

Little did I know that when it came time to search for work, the baby boom generation would hit the workplace, making it impossible to find a job teaching English. If only I hadn't inherited the double anxiety genes of panic disorder. It took away most of my choices, I thought. Who would marry me? A foreigner, perhaps, desperate enough for US citizenship? Maybe a man like that would love me enough to take care of me. I grew up on Cinderella.

Only the Prince Charming types went for the girls whose dads could set them up in business. I didn't look like Cinderella. I looked like Woody Allen, with a high IQ to match. Sometimes smart gals make really dumb mistakes in their choice of men. What did I learn? That however far you travel to find the right man, you end up with a man just like your dear old dad in personality.

I did—twice. Now I fumed at the thought that a high-school dropout girl who looked like Gina Lollobrigida, an Italian American friend of mine married a wealthy Jewish lawyer from a family that owned a private house in Long Island. And not only didn't he beat her; he hired a maid for her. They ended up with three children, a 4,000 square foot private house with a big backyard, and I ended up homeless and penniless. Who took away my choices? My genes made my destiny? I couldn't let that happen.

Persistence and determination were my best two qualities. It was that certain stubbornness to go to any extreme to get attention that some men detested. What I kept were diaries. I read my mom's diary: "October 26, 1926, first day of my honeymoon: today I died." I tried on her white satin wedding shoes, size four with high heel pumps and short, matching satin wedding dress circa 1926, well preserved. The dress didn't age. She did. The shoes were too small for my size nine feet. The dress fit.

I couldn't fill my mom's shoes without spilling over. I filled my dad's shoes, but the thought made me feel uneasy. My greatest gift to myself was my oceanic personality. I had to get away from angry men. Yet I married one angry husband after another. Why? Each time I married it was right after losing my job, the only shield that separated me from being a homeless shopping bag lady at any age.

When I rushed over to Darlene's house, she fully intended to confide everything in her best friend. Darlene was her analyst and confessor. What else are best girl friends for? Darlene let I bring her dates to her luscious home.

When we double dated, Darlene would go off in one living room to make out on the couch with her date and turn off the light, leaving me to the other living room couch in the dark with my own date to talk about how awkward we felt trying to remain friendly when I put distance between us for the sake of protecting my own health. That was friendship. This time I confided one too many with Darlene. She arrived in the early afternoon and used the great gold lion knocker on the mahogany door.

"What's the emergency now?" Darlene was surprised I would show up on a school day. We sat opposite each other on Darlene's white suede sofa.

Darlene couldn't wait to get in her latest news. "I met this bald guy at Grossinger's. He's twenty-nine, a pharmacist. But I had to let him go. There's no way he could ever support me the way my dad does."

Darlene was the epitome of the Jewish American Princess, the German Jewish uptown princess that I fantasized about, envied and admired. Darlene was the Blue Book Jewess whose family had been in America since before 1830. Society.

It didn't even dawn on me that my own heritage might be even more unique. All I could think of to blurt out to Darlene was "My mom has been arrested for shoplifting."

Darlene sat across from me and stared for a long while without saying anything. She handed me a bowl of peanuts.

"And my brother's the lawyer defending my mom."

Benjamin, my brother, had graduated from law school in 1956 and was a starving lawyer trying to get into real estate. "Law is not for poor boys," he always said.

"I don't think I can ever leave my parent's home," Darlene said, not even responding to my amazing true confession.

"Don't you understand how I feel now that my mom's been arrested for shoplifting? I repeated.

"Would you trade this house for independence and a roach-filled studio apartment in the Village?" Darlene seemed wrapped up in her own thoughts.

"I'm so ashamed of being ashamed," I sobbed. "She was nabbed with a flimsy nightie in a way too-small size-my size-draped over her arm. I've been telling her to stop since I was seven. I couldn't touch those things. They're evil. Doesn't she see boundaries between herself and somebody else's stuff?" I tried to explain how I felt to Darlene, but she tuned me out.

"My psychotherapist is waiting. I really do have an appointment now." Darlene added.

She got up and motioned for me to leave. "A sexy nightie?" Darlene added, looking back at I over her shoulder.

"It was a petite size. But my mom weighs more than two hundred-fifty pounds and is only five feet tall. She kept saying she forgot the thing was hanging over her shoulder."

As Darlene walked toward the door with me following, she began to laugh loudly and inappropriately. "This will crack up my analyst. You've got to be crazy to see a psychiatrist nowadays."

I continued to ramble even though Darlene had already checked out. "When she walked out the door of the department store, she was in a daze from her high blood pressure pills. The security guard tackled her, knocking her to the ground, smashing her head against the pavement."

"What you need is to sue the store. Why don't you call my dad?"

I sighed. "My brother is a lawyer."

"How could a man tackle an old woman?" Darlene squinted at me in disbelief.

"I don't know who to believe anymore. Did my mom really take it or did she really forget?"

Darlene walked me down the driveway and to her bus stop. "We've been having terrible security problems with our sliding glass door. How's that Syrian boyfriend of yours?"

I beamed at her best girlfriend. "We're getting married October twenty-fifth."

"Oh?" Darlene's face drooped in a jealous rage. She looked sideways and up toward the clouds, giggling. "I had a Lebanese lover once. We both were seventeen. He was a Maronite Catholic I met in prep school."

"It must have ended pretty gruesome."

Darlene flushed with anger. "His parents forbid him to see me. Sex can be beautiful if it's with someone who knows what he's doing."

"Darlene, I have no one else to be my sister." "I can't ever really be your sister," Darlene shot back. "My own sister just finished her doctorate. She's a famous screenwriter out in Los Angeles. And I'm nothing. Nothing without her. That's why I need another sister like a dolphin needs a mink coat."

"I came over to tell you I'm getting married," I hawked. "And to get some sympathy for my mom."

"Don't marry your boyfriend. Find yourself a nice, Jewish boy."

"But nice, Jewish boys are not interested in me. I don't have the rich, observant family to back me up. My mother is from a Jewish family. The clean-cut, employed Jewish architect, doctor, lawyer, Washington FBI agent, science professor, or stockbroker type I'd want to marry wants a princess. So far when I met that type he always asked 'What does your father do for a living?' Nobody ever asked me what I do for a living, what I'm studying or what I want to do.

"It's glossed over as if it's unimportant. Well it's important to me. It's all I have, my personality and my future potential as a professional somewhere. My father mops toilets in the Navy yard at night when he is able to work, and when his nerves don't get the best of him. My mom's a housewife because she's too old and sick to be a maid in a beauty parlor any more. I'm not rich or loved enough to attract a prince. I don't even have the big boobs or the trust fund. What I need is drastic change to be happy."

"The Arab is drastic change," Darlene shook her head and smirked. "But you won't be happy. He'll treat you differently than he'd treat a woman from his own country. He won't treat you as if Arabs and Jews were once the same people. He'll treat you the same as he'd treat a Swedish or German lady—as a temporary piece of ass in a foreign country."

"He kisses his mother's hand and touches her hand to forehead. If he respects her, he'll respect me, too."

"No he won't. You're an outsider, an American whom his culture sees as a foreign whore. And you've never asked his mother how often her husband beats her."

For a moment my mind flashed back on the word "whore." By habit, father always called me a tramp.

"What will you do the first time you fight and he calls you a dirty Jew or spits in your face?" Darlene stopped in her tracks.

"Rich, educated Jewish boys won't marry flat-chested girls with hook noses and scars on their chins or poor fathers." I stuck out my tongue.

"Look," I added, "My dad's a janitor, an eighth-grade dropout. My mom left school in the fifth grade. I'm a straight-A university student who put myself through one hundred percent, working in the library. Don't you think I deserve a good provider, an intelligent man?"

"No!" Darlene insisted.

"You have no divine right to any man. It's sheer luck. Some women just don't have the script in their head that they deserve a good man. If the script's not there, they can't be looking for a good provider. They only run to the excitement."

"With a father like mine, what kind of a man would I go for? Darlene, I can't afford your therapist."

"Go to a classy synagogue. Give your future kids a chance."

"When they meet my folks, they'll leave!" I persisted. "Do you know what synagogue memberships cost?"

"Your college has no men?"

"My courses are filled with women majoring in poetry writing, most are in the same little cliques, one for each ethnic group, and all with engagement rings-doctor's daughters and daughters of vice presidents of big corporations. I found an Armenian and a Greek friend who are outsiders like me. I'm an outsider only because I'm poor and have no connections. Maybe I need to join more associations, but those professional associations cost money."

"And at work?"

"The single ones are uneducated shipping clerks. The older men are married."

"And you think I enjoy getting date-raped by doctors at Grossingers?" Darlene groaned. "Last time it was a short red-haired lawyer who wouldn't drive me home unless he parked under a bridge."

"And they know your dad is a judge?" I screeched.

"What about the dances at the Law Schools?"

I complained, "Every time a guy asked me to dance the first question out of his mouth was 'What does your father do for a living?' I told him he mops toilets at night in the Navy Yard as a general laborer for a hundred bucks a week."

"If I can't find a stable, Jewish husband at Grossingers at those prices, I guess you'll have to settle. But I won't." Darlene waved goodbye, leaving me at her bus stop. She unlocked her white Mercedes-Benz.

"Don't they even care to ask what I do for a living?" I called to her. "Isn't it good enough my brother worked his way through law school working as a bookkeeper? He even earned his CPA."

As Darlene slid into the red plush seat she snickered, "Your prince wouldn't want you to work and neglect his babies. With your luck for misers, you wouldn't get a maid."

My bus arrived and she stepped out. "Do quality men freak out when a girl's mother visits relatives who are storefront gypsies for psychic reading? Are all women judged by the profession of the men they marry, in spite of how creative they are, how many books they write, or how many university degrees they have?" The bus driver looked at me like I was nuts.

"What are you looking at?" I told the driver. "Didn't you ever see a Jewish-nisha evil eye before?"

That night, I sat in my room thinking about all that had happened since my mom had returned home from Florida, unwillingly, having run out of money. How she hated having to come back to the roach-infested Brooklyn apartment.

As I read an archaeology book, the phone rang. I ran to the foyer to answer it. There was only one phone and it was centrally located on my brother's desk in the foyer, a desk made from a kitchen table painted black and covered by oil cloth.

It was Darlene on the other end, sounding hopeless. "My $125 real leather purse is missing, I. I'm giving you a chance to return it before I call the insurance company."

I couldn't believe what I heard. "You must be nuts. I didn't take your purse. Such a thing is totally against every fiber of my being."

"My mother's on the extension, listening," Darlene said.

"Please, please go back to your therapist. It's not worth our friendship to ruin my reputation," I begged. "Don't betray me like this just because I'm marrying that Syrian guy and you can't fall in love."

"You have one chance to return my purse," Darlene said coldly.

"Damn it! I didn't take anything. Why the hell did you tell your mother what I told you in confidence?" The idea of taking anything to me is disgusting. It violates boundaries. I know what it feels like to find someone has taken money from my purse. Now my friend had betrayed me, another loss. I had confided in her, and she made up lies. Why did people with money have to be so cruel to me? And why did I want to be so much like them as far as having money? I turned to studying irony to find an answer from my books on irony in classical philosophy, but I really needed practical answers I could apply to life.

On a separate line Darlene's famous artist mother, Goldie dialed up Benjamin. My brother had worked late at his law office.

"Listen to this," Goldie announced. She got Benjamin on the line. "I hear your mother was arrested for shoplifting. What kind of a lawyer are you anyway? I'll see to it that you're disbarred now that your sister stole my daughter's expensive purse."

"I don't have to answer to such trash." Benjamin's voice went tense and high-pitched. She had gotten him by the balls and now was whirling him around like a pin-wheel.

Benjamin hung up on her, but I hung on for dear life, afraid to cut the cord, wanting so much a relationship that I was willing to compete for it.

"If you can't trust your best friend, who do you trust with your life when your family goes to pieces?"

"Didn't you hear my mother on the phone?" Darlene insisted. "I know you took it. No one else was there."

"Darlene, why are you so jealous of my boyfriend? You think he's some rich sheik?"

"My daughter never lies," Goldie answered now on the third extension line.

"Just because you keep breaking up with your own boyfriends? Because you lost your Lebanese lover? What gives you the right to revenge in your innocent friend?" I sobbed.

"If you don't return my daughter's purse, I'm going to take action against you." Goldie had lost all patience.

"Just because your first real boyfriend's Lebanese family rejected your Jewish background for their son, Darlene, there's no reason to make up lies to put me down in order to build yourself up. You'd go to any extreme to get your mom's attention.

"Maybe you don't have the confidence to compete with your younger sister. So you're spending on me all that anger you've banked for her and your mom. She's beautiful, has the graduate degree currently in demand, and a dream job most people wish for in their prayers. And she's your mother's favorite. I understand that you feel unimportant when you compare your unemployment, your looks, and college dropout background to your younger sister's achievements." I was grasping at anything. "Maybe if we both talked to your therapist at your next appointment, I can find out why you lied to get your mom's attention and at the same time victimized me. Isn't it enough I have to deal with my dad's raging temper without my best friend using me as a scapegoat?

Darlene sighed with frustration. "That purse was expensive. I bought it for one hundred twenty-five dollars in Antigua, damn it."

"People like you shouldn't be coming to our house," Goldie nagged. I heard you're marrying a Muslim. All your kids will be forced to grow up Arab Muslim."

"Listen you overbearing mother, you can't control my life. I'm not your emotionally disturbed kid in therapy."

I seemed to be talking specifically to her mother, to all universal archetype mothers in general, to all authority figures.

"I pity you," Darlene insisted. "That's why you must bring it back right away."

"You trashed your own purse. Why do you feel the need to hurt me? Am I your victim? And everybody attacks the same victim? Is asking for help a sign of weakness?"

"Bring back the purse in the morning or else the insurance investigators will be on your tail."

"You must be miserable, Darlene. Is that why you're in therapy? I'm getting married next month, and I'm graduating from college and succeeding. You can't stand in my way."

Goldie's voice poured its hot lead. "The insurance company will make a lot of trouble for your brother's law practice."

"Goldie, you're a bitter old lady." When I got mad, she got verbal. She analyzed. "And Darlene, was it because you dropped out of college? Or are your afraid to move out of your parent's house? Or maybe this is the way you're getting at your younger sister because she won a fellowship. Why use me as your younger sister? A new punching pillow? Can't you talk to your real sister?"

Darlene overreacted with violent noises. "You have the problem, sister." She was stifling herself ladylike.

"You've never confided in me, Darlene. Not the way I've opened up to you. I've given you too much power over me. By God, it must be something you hate in yourself. Now I know the rich aren't all happy-just comfortably sick. I banged the receiver down with a vengeance.

9

October 25, 1963: Our Wedding Day

I brought Ahmed into the Syrian synagogue. The first thing that hit him was the scent of orange blossoms and incense that wafted through the atrium.

"Smells and looks just like a mosque," he said.

Ahmed turned this way and that. I noticed how his smiling green eyes turned down at the corners in a crude way, making him appear much older than his twenty-six years.

He stepped into the office and talked in Arabic with one of the rabbis. I didn't notice who said what, only that the conversation wasn't in English. I waited by the doorway, almost afraid to set foot in an intensely male dominated setting. It was something I consciously sought, a darling daddy so I could be daddy's darling.

When Ahmed came out, he told me that the rabbi said a big wedding in the synagogue would cost about ten thousand dollars. I was shocked and disappointed. It was my life-long wish to be married in a big ceremony in an exotic, Sephardic synagogue-anywhere, even if I had to drag in the only man I felt I could attract-a foreigner in desperate need of an American passport. What other man would want the likes of unlovable I? I thought.

There was always that ghostly lover, that fantasy that could never be real. I dreamed of an unreal lover, one I created who lived in her imagination more than three hundred years ago. The man I loved was burned at the stake for Judaizing in the great auto de fe of 1649 in Mexico city, and I could never hope to recapture this former life, not there, nor here, nor in the Seville I came from in that former life.

But there was Ahmed in the here and now. There could never be Avy Joseph, the incarnation of the one soulmate of my past life, I dreamed, even though I was standing in the very place where he was bar mitzvah when they both were thirteen in 1955.

I dragged the Syrian Muslim Ahmed into the Syrian Jewish synagogue. I made him promise he'd go through with a Jewish ceremony for her. Perhaps to him it was worth an American passport five years down the line. It was the only way, I felt, when one wasn't good enough for a real Jewish prince.

There were shortages of princes for average girls without money, pedigree, or technical graduate degrees. But the movies allowed daydreams.

Dreams don't ever die. I reasoned that maybe the rabbi would marry them cheaply in his office if only Ahmed asked. But Ahmed couldn't tell the rabbi his first name was Ahmed. That's a Muslim name.

Ahmed left on friendly terms. I never knew exactly what conversation went on between them in Arabic. It didn't even occur to me, hopelessly lost in my dreams, that no Syrian rabbi would marry a Muslim to a Jew knowingly, and that Ahmed's name would never be taken for Jewish unless he changed it outright to a Jewish name.

At that point, Ahmed took control. He whisked me from the synagogue and took me to where one of his Arab friends who had lived in the U.S. for years suggested: the city clerk's office.

Instead of the Sephardic synagogue, the great Spanish and Portuguese one in New York, where I felt I belonged, I was married in a civil ceremony by the city clerk.

It was a legal ceremony, devoid of any religious tract. "A drastic change is necessary for happiness," I told Ahmed. "If Jews treated me so badly, how will Arabs receive me?

"You need witnesses," the clerk told Ahmed. I had managed to go through college without making even one close friend. I enjoyed being a loner. Ahmed had all the friends, other Arab immigrants trying to make ends meet.

Sociophobia, fear of people, was my middle name. All I had received from people was trouble. As a movie buff, I had spent all her spare time studying film-women in film, documentaries. I lived for the travel films but was afraid to fly or even to leave the city.

I never told my parents when I married. Two witnesses were finally dug up from Ahmed's acquaintances he made in the six weeks he had been in New York-his English teacher and a male buddy from another Arab country.

Not until after the ceremony and the short, Dutch-treat lunch of chicken chow mein in a Brooklyn restaurant with the two witnesses, did I and Ahmed return to her parent's apartment to tell them.

Why didn't I invite her parents to her wedding? Meyer's remarks were perpetually withholding of love, money, flattery, praise, and kindness. Tsipke represented to I the eternal victim, the Diaspora of one. The very fact that Tsipke stood with Meyer all these years, taking it in the belly, too weak to move, too sacrificing and complaining about it angered I. For every moment of self imprisonment Tsipke would blame the baby of the family-I. It was I who caused all Tsipke's ills. If it weren't for her, there would be a divorce. "I've only stayed for the sake of the children."

I was the only child around who couldn't ever grow. "Why 'd you stay and then hate me for making you stay with my father?" I would ask her mother.

"Why succumb for my sake?" All that on my shoulders. Dump the pain on I. The buck stopped here. I was expected to absorb her mother's stress like a bottomless well.

No sooner did I withdraw sixty dollars of her college loan money to pay for a honeymoon night at the Americana hotel, than did I find out that as I was getting married, President Kennedy was getting shot. It ruined the romance of her honeymoon night.

Right after the marriage I found out through Ahmed's friend, the interpreter, that my new husband was not a doctor of mechanical engineering at all. He was really a high-school dropout without even a diploma who went to Germany to learn how to be a machinist in a factory. That's what he did for a living-machinist work in factories. Ahmed was out of a job, had no American experience as a machinist, was totally out of money now, and dependent on me.

I gave him three dollars a day from my college loan money to take the subway to find work each morning. The marriage night was painful.

When I finally dashed back to see my parents after the wedding and before going to the hotel for the night, mom-Tsipke rushed downstairs to the pharmacy and bought a gift-wrapped package of condoms.

The box was all done up with ribbons and fancy wrapping paper. Ahmed ripped it open thinking it was an expensive wedding present from my parents. He laughed when he found out it was only some old rubbers.

"I didn't want you to get pregnant on your wedding night," Tsipke giggled, taking a pigeon-toed stance. On a sixty-year old fat woman with blue-black hair and transparent silver eyes, the girlish giggling didn't look cute anymore, only matronly.

Ahmed looked over his new mother-in-law. I wasn't even surprised or concerned when I told her they were already married that afternoon. Meyer nodded and left the room after looking Ahmed up and down. Only last week Meyer had chased him from the house for staying too late and he was the only fellow to come back. Pretty desperate for that American green card, I thought. Why else would any man want her, I reasoned.

Before dinner, I had shelled out three dollars to Ahmed from college loan money. It slipped away quickly, and I still had eight weeks to go until graduation.

By six in the evening, Ahmed and I rode the subway toward the America Hotel in Manhattan. At once I realized that I had married a 26-year old failure, and that I became a loser, someone who wouldn't "make it" in life. I had always thought myself as a creative person who must express creativity and share it with others, inspire and motivate others as I created along with the world, but after five years of college, with a master's degree in creative writing and English switched from a visual anthropology major about finished now, I thought—don't I deserve a good man, too? Must a twenty-two year old woman settle only to find someone to pay the rent so I could continue studying until I had a doctorate and became an academic?

A failure, a schmuck, a putz, a jerk, a schlemiel, a dib (bear) in Arabic is a victim and a receiver. A deeb in Arabic is a wolf who's clever enough to hang around humans to get scraps of food. Any man who'd ride the subway to his honeymoon hotel must be a failure, I thought. But of course, any woman who was afraid to learn to drive deserved a man who was a failure. And any woman who'd have him deserved the same fate.

I knew at gut level he would never be the good provider I most desperately wanted. At the same time I couldn't understand why dad always called me a tramp and then said that he feared I'd become a tramp and be 'trouble.' Why would a 21-year old virgin college student be called a tramp simply for wanting to be married and settled?

In New York City, 1963, finding a marriage-minded 'date' for me meant paying a computer dating service. I did. And the few men sent my way never called back. One was a physicist. I would have liked to talk with him again. The other was a PhD in foreign languages and psychology who taught at a university and traveled.

He would have been a good conversationalist. I know I never had a wedding and never had a honeymoon or a vacation lasting more than one or two days. I would have liked all those things. What I got instead was travel videos and what-if daydreams. What if there's no next life to meet my soul mate, my intended, my *beshert*? What if my soul mate beats me because the soup was tepid? Does that mean he's not my soul mate after all?

At that moment I knew I would never be family because I never really had family, not loving family. This was the script I carried inside. I looked over at Ahmed. What was his script, I wondered? Everybody has a script that says something is important.

In the hotel room he put on the condom and rammed it into me dry. The pain was excruciating. He was a premature ejaculator and couldn't last more than one stroke. He never changed. To me, even sex was more bullshit, and I never felt anything from it except panic disorder. At that moment I realized in a former life I could have been Emily Dickenson, but probably was not.

At this point, reason and logic seemed so harmonious in preference to feelings and I had to step out of feelings like an athlete shedding sweaty underwear. Reason, solving intricate mathematical problems seemed to wash me clean.... clean as Laplace transformations and chaos theory.

In the morning, I unpacked his suitcase when out fell a bunch of love letters written in German. I had studied three foreign languages in college. I was able to read enough of the letters to translate that a girl in Germany had borne Ahmed's baby girl and had written to him in Syria a love letter. One line read, "How can you leave your own flesh and blood? How can you deny this baby is yours?"

When Ahmed woke, I asked him who is this woman? Why did he run back to Syria, away from his own child? "Ah, the woman is a whore," Ahmed told I. "But how can you leave your flesh and blood?"

"It's not my baby, he insisted. "Besides, you think I'd marry a Nazi whore-a German woman, after what the Germans did in the War? You think my father would let me marry a German who slept with men before me?"

"How about a Jew?" I inquired.

"A Jew is like an Arab. You look like a woman from the Middle East. Besides, you were a virgin."

"I still am."

I gave him back his German letters and let it go. "I wonder what the baby looks like?" After three months of marriage, the fights began. Already, I wanted to leave. I enrolled for a PhD in cinema research and writing, and got pregnant just before dissertation time. I never did go back to finish at that school. Years later I earned a Masters degree in creative writing/English at the age of forty.

◆   ◆   ◆

10

August 1964—The Train Ride In New Jersey: Disguised As An Arab Housewife In A Brooklyn Jewish Neighborhood For Nearly Seven Years

Ahmed and I returned from a vacation in Asbury Park, New Jersey. I had taken Ahmed to stay at one of the many Syrian Jewish hotels in Bradley Beach, where single Syrian Jews customarily went to find marriage partners before Deal, New Jersey became the matchmaker's paradise and Brooklyn housed most of the community.

It was one of the hottest August 1964 days as the train rushed back to New York. I was two-months pregnant. I had my medium dark ash brown hair dyed blue-back and curled into an Egyptian style. My eyes were made up to look like Liz Taylor in the 1964 hit of "Cleopatra."

For some time now I was disguising myself as an Arab woman married to an Arab man in New York-if only to see what it feels like being an Arab in a Jewish ghetto. Once in journalism class, a professor began to bark about how the Arabs wouldn't let him teach in Lebanon because he was a Jew.

He was in shock when I told him my Arab husband's name and later dropped out of the class. He put down the Lebanese and ranted in anger at Arabs for rejecting him as a Jew, giving back the treatment he had received as a university teacher in Lebanon.

Then when I interviewed for a publishing job, I was hired and then called back and told I would not be wanted at that company solely because my resume mentioned that I was the wife of an "Arab sheik." Later, I published my writing in a major New York-based magazine and won many awards in college for short stories.

It was fun posing as an Arab woman among Jews, getting the brunt of the discrimination that had for so long been dumped on me for looking "Jewish" (Semitic) in this case.

However, it was no fun getting beaten to hell by a neo-Nazi for simply looking Jewish and not obeying. After a two-day vacation at a plush, Syrian Jewish boarding house hotel in Bradley Beach, the train headed toward Elizabeth, New Jersey on its way to Manhattan. In one train car I sat with my mother who had vacationed in her own room with my husband and myself at our expense. Ahmed* (name changed for privacy) was in a good mood this month because he was working.

I had to get up to go to the john that required passing between train cars. As I tried to come back from the rest room and pass again between the cars to get back to her seat, a man suddenly blocked her way.

He had a face out of a Norman Rockwell print. American gothic. Balding black hair, round blue eyes with thick glasses. A face like Hitler, but tall and thin. His wife stood inside the car a few feet from him, with the breeze hitting her. Pillbox hat and fishnet veil, blue cotton dress, dark brown hair and squinty brown eyes. The couple was in their early fifties, maybe late forties.

"Wait 'till the train stops," the well-dressed man in a gray suit commanded.

"But I've got to get back to my seat or my husband will worry that I became sick in the john," I whined.

Here I was two months pregnant, twenty-two, morning sickness, and with black-and-blue arms from a recent blood test at the OB office the day before.

The man shook his head "no." But I, not about to give a strange man that much power over me, rushed past him as if I refused to have space in my life for people like him. For once, I thought, having read that book called *The Feminine Mystique*, that I could get away with being treated in a crowded public train in the afternoon as a majority male.

The American gothic male grabbed my face and wrestled me down so that my head was between his knees. He began to crush my skull sideways between his thighs in a vise-like grip. Then he took his knee and squeezed my head between the metal of the inside train car and his leg. Like a rag doll, he twisted me, grabbing lifting my flailing body upwards and putting it down inside the car.

I tried to run in place like a fool, but he was holding me steadfast while my legs circled as if pumping a bicycle.

"Let her go dear," came a child like tone from his wife. She only spoke openly when she saw my outstretched arm flailing and my wiggling fingers with that bright gold wedding band flashing in the woman's eye.

Once the woman saw my wedding ring, all sorts of things could have flashed before her. Perhaps she realized that there may be a hunk of a husband lurking in the next car. Her voice whispered.

"Let her go, dear."

The age fifty-something man, goyisha-looking (American Gothic-Norman Rockwell painting lookalike) let me go at last, but not before he gave me a swift kick at the base of the spine and threw me forward, bodily into the next car. With that, he yelled to me, "You dirty Jew!" and then a stream of epithets.

Not one of the other passengers rose to my aid.

No one cared to get involved or even look up from their newspapers.

When you look sixteen, men don't spare the rod. I thought. If he knew I was twenty-two, married, and pregnant, would he have done it the same way? Probably, I wondered.

I trotted back to my seat in dead silence and never told my husband what happened and never told mother, either.

What if I had said something? I wondered. My husband would get into a fight. It wouldn't be good for the baby to continue the tension. So for the rest of my life, I kept silent on this event.

Except, once I even wrote a letter to the editor of the newspaper in Elizabeth, where the man might have gotten off. All I knew was that that man in the train told me to wait until the train stopped before passing him. Why that hullabaloo merely to return to my seat from the john? All that punching and painful head squeezing against a metal wall, all for a 119 pound, five foot-four pregnant lady. Forget morning sickness on a two-day vacation. It's a train's passenger who beat me up. No one rose to help or even looked up from their newspapers. I didn't make a sound but waved my wedding ring at the man's wife.

How'd he know I was Jewish? I wondered, looking at my face in a compact mirror. I could have been anything: Armenian, Spanish, Italian, Greek, Arab, Welsh, Yugoslavian, French, Swiss, Persian, Austrian, or a mix of everything Adriatic. I went through naming all the countries I could pass as natives of. Why be called a dirty Jew from a stranger on a train? Was he really a neo Nazi or what? Could this only happen where there were many Jews living side by side with an area in which Jews were kept out by anti-Semitic gangs? What did he have against pregnant Jewish women?

Was I too pushy? Perhaps the dark hair and convex nose sparked some fatal anger in him. How did he know I wasn't Welsh? After all, British people have hook noses and black hair with white, freckled skin, like me and olive green eyes. In 1964 there weren't that many Iranians around, so there was that less to choose from. I could have been Sicilian or even Irish.

Why did he see a convex nose and black hair, and suddenly start to beat me up with a rage I saw in my dad all the time. Now a strange man on a train exploded at me. When would I find a man slow to anger with kindness where I could feel safe sitting next to him? Where could I find peace and serenity? In what occupation or place?

Only five years ago I get in a bus and a blonde young man asks me where am I from, Israel? That's in San Diego. I blurted, "Portugal" but I could have said "Soviet Georgia or Abkhazia on the Black Sea, or any other unique place. The stereotype came out of his mouth before I said a word. Why jump to a conclusion and then explode volcanically with bigotry to a stranger in a bus with whom he wanted to make conversation.

Back in 1964 in the train, all that I did was what any red-blooded American male would do as his right. How could my passing in front of him offended? Was disobeying his word enough to set him off just because I was a Jewish-looking woman-a black-haired woman with pale, freckled skin and a hook nose? Should I have obeyed him?

Then I'd have to take it from my husband who commanded me to listen only to his orders? If a woman doesn't belong to one man, is she the property of all men? Must all women obey all men or die? Why do men explode in hostility at a stereotypical 'Jewish' face as if there really had been such a caricature. What's the difference between an ancient Roman or Greek face and a Levantine face? Nothing. I thought and thought again. It's the litmus test of man's humanity to the strange woman perceived to be alone on the street, in a bus, or on a train.

◆   ◆   ◆

11

September 1964: Who Turned On The Gas Jets?

One night in my third month of pregnancy I awoke to find that someone had turned on all the gas jets in my basement Brooklyn apartment. Was it my husband? Did he want to get rid of me? Or did a stranger come downstairs? Was it the family from whom we rented a tiny basement apartment in their duplex? Why? There was no motive.

Who turned on all the gas in the middle of the night? I awoke because of the smell, went into the dark kitchen, lit a light, and noticed all the gas jets were going full blast without the pilot light. Someone had to have gotten up in the night and turned them on while I slept.

The day before, Ahmed had received his green card, and now was able to legally work in America. My parents, my brother, and I no longer supported him, but I needed evidence that he was trying to kill me. Perhaps he couldn't quite make up his mind if he wanted to go through with it.

The day before I went to the hospital in March 1965 to have my daughter, Ahmed got into the savings passbook.

"Where's all the money?" His hazel eyes burned with evil.

"I spent it for food."

"The whole six hundred dollars?"

"If you weren't pregnant, I'd put my fist through your belly button," he shouted.

A year later when I told him I was pregnant with our son, he said, "Get rid of it." However, when the baby was born, he wanted it so much, he sent it overseas to his mother in Syria to raise against my cries, and spit in my face, pulled my hair, and chased me a block with a restaurant carving knife.

Just like dad, "If I catch you, I'll kill you," rang in my ears once again. In my second marriage, my German-English husband chased me through the alley as I screamed, "Wife beater," and he paced agitated wallowing in his own sense of inadequacy, not able to keep his hands off my neck.

Why do the men I meet want to kill me? Why did my dad tell me over and over he wanted to flush me down the toilet? Why did he try to kill me? Why did the nine-year old Italian American neighbor boy invite me when I, too was nine, into his backyard to play with his pet rabbits and then piss on me, laughing as he soiled me? Roman Justice?

Someday will a man in my life or a man that I meet as stranger outside strangle me, perhaps because I'm old and frail? Yesterday a teenager passing angrily yelled at me, "Old Lady." He thought I was looking at him on his skateboard as I tried to walk by him to reach the mailbox.

Why did the man crossing the street scream at me on my sixty-first birthday and use the words "Dirty Jew?" What made them assume I'm Jewish, let alone use the term 'dirty' as I'm clean and well dressed and look like any teacher or professional woman or even most secretaries or librarians?

I have Mars in Aries in my seventh house of partnerships square my Venus in Capricorn, the love sign, in my fourth house of domesticity, denoting friction and violence from the husband. Many years ago my husband tried to strangle me several times always stopping short with a beet-red face, biting his tongue in anger to get power, as I ran out of the house, and then he calmed down.

He had an explosive temper and still took phenylaniline in a health food supplement because someone told him it was good for an aging brain. Penniless as usual, I always have had no where to go, no money to pay rent, no income, and had no job in thirty years.

As a vegetarian and health-food connoisseur, I take no drugs, never smoke, and eat a balanced diet. For health's sake I take fish oils or add fish to my diet now and then. I do my Yoga exercises, Qi Gong, and Tai Chi for balance as a senior. Why is life for little old ladies so unsafe? Why are old people so lonely and friends so difficult to find? And why are the young who befriend the old so readily interested in stealing their cash? Where is love when you're old? Answers arrive when I exercise with the chi energy in the air, the life force in everything that grows in nature.

Back in 1965, when I was twenty-three and a graduate student, Ahmed would drift from job to job, always picking fights with his supervisor and getting fired. He was running out of places to work in New York as a machinist.

"Ahmed has gone nuts, just like my dad," I would phone mother. There was something in his eyes that I couldn't read. But it had triumph in it.

We didn't have any medical insurance. As a foreigner, Ahmed didn't know such things existed. His job didn't offer any benefits. He wasn't on a job much longer than three months anyway, before he was fired for trouble with his boss or lack of skills. Ahmed never learned to read or write English. He'd watch television and then ask me to read the newspaper to him aloud.

"How'd you two ever get together?" Mrs. Feinstein, a neighbor woman, once asked me, seeing my first husband around. "You two don't look like you'd ever have anything in common. I mean, you, a frail intellectual ghetto type. And him, a hulking man of no class, refinement, or education. How come?" I should have said because we both had inferiority complexes, deep senses of inadequacy. Instead, I looked for outward reasons.

"He was the first man who wanted me. He lied. He told me that he was a doctor of mechanical engineering." In reality, he was a secondary school dropout and a machinist in German factories.

"So why stay?"

"All I wanted was a successful financial man, a stockbroker, mutual fund company CFO or technical financial analyst type to enjoy buying and selling stocks and talking about mutual funds. Or maybe I wanted a professor of anthropology and nutrition? Or a psychiatrist who is deeply religious, but not punitive and judgmental? My mom's half sister's daughter married a psychiatrist and has a fantastic, huge house in the palm latitudes. She's never invited me to her home.

When I visited her once, she excused herself to go out with friends on a weekend afternoon. All I wanted to do was walk through her home once and marvel proudly. That's my niece. But she never invited me because I married poor. She works as a volunteer now and then in a skilled nursing home for the aged. As a doctor's wife she thinks she's better than me. She doesn't know my son is a doctor, too. And I have a similar college degree just like her.

That's what I call rejection by family. Why do relatives appear so cold, stern, and distant? I've created family newsletters and tried to keep in touch, but being old and invisible, they don't communicate because there's little they think I can do for them financially. Their wealth will go to their own children, of course. But while I am here, I can't understand why they won't be pen pals. Yes. I do understand. Youth is busy working 80 hours a week. We retirees need to stick together to test that bromide of too much time on our hands and too little money that pays homage to the clock.

Why would a successful man look twice at me-in spite of five years of college? What man would want a woman who keeps going to pieces if not cherished like a princess? I have nothing more to give. My body can't take one more punch. Would a successful man want that?"

"What do you really want?

"A man to take care of me like the prince took care of Cinderella but without being controlling. I want to be a Jewish American Princess to one man-without being punished and beaten by those who hate Jews just for looking Jewish or Middle Eastern peoples for looking Middle Eastern or looking South Asian.

"I want a daddy to love me and a mommy to say I love you instead of I never wanted you, but I'm taking care of you only because it's my job, like my mom said. I want parents who didn't tell me they wanted to flush me down the toilet or a mom who didn't say she got pregnant because her father paid her a visit and she had to sleep for once in the same bedroom as her own husband so her dad could have a room to himself."

"Can't a woman with a university master's degree in liberal arts get a good job?"

"I won't teach because I'm afraid to speak in public. And I hate secretarial work. There's no way I can support myself, let alone children. Without a man I can wake up in the morning knowing I'm still alive. On the other hand, I'm nothing without a man to pay the bills, I told Mrs. Feinstein.

"Oh," Mrs. Feinstein sighed, and went back to her own family. "I'm only like you on the inside." The morning I went in to have her baby, I had a fight with Ahmed. I took the subway alone to the hospital. When I told the admitting clerk I was alone, another woman sitting and waiting in the office to have her baby looked at me with a cold, dark-eyed stare and so did her husband standing beside her. Probably they thought I was single.

All the other couples were there together. Two hours of mild menstrual cramps, a caudal with the first baby, an epidural block with the second that numbs from the waist down, no pain, only reading the comic books, forgetting trouble, enjoying the experience of birth compared to living day to day in the marriage.

Three hours later the baby was born, easy case, simple labor. I felt so relaxed from the two Nembutals that as they wheeled me into the delivery room I sat up on one elbow and smiled, "I feel like I'm relaxing on a sunny beach." It was great compared to being a battered wife at home and listening to the put-downs my two men in '65 or '76 used to build themselves up using me as a verbal or literal punching bag.

Too bad I had the choice taken away not to have an unnecessary episiotomy. The stitches kept me constipated for two weeks. I got pregnant again right away after I told my husband I didn't want any more children. One February morning I had the flu, and thought I wouldn't get pregnant right after my period, but I did.

He told me to get rid of it. I didn't. As soon as the second baby was born, the agoraphobia came back twice as strong as it felt after the first child. This time the fear returned with white-outs in the bus and tremors.

The first, a girl, was born at four in the afternoon. Ahmed came to visit and took charge of *his* baby. I had lost "possession" of my daughter already. The talk about sending the baby to Syria had started. So soon I became invisible.

I never forgot I was now a battered wife like mom. He had started to beat me while I was pregnant. Now I felt for sure he had tried to murder her by turning on the gas jets and then changed his mind. Later, when I married my second husband, I found out he had the same personality type as my dad—ISFJ on the Myers-Briggs Type Indicator, a popular personality test.

Not only did I marry twice, two men that treated me like my father treated mom and me, but I married someone with the identical personality type. My first marriage was to an Arab Muslim and my second to an Anglo-Saxon Protestant, and in each case, I married a man so much like my dad, even though I went to the extreme to marry different ethnic groups and religions from my own father.

Still, I couldn't break away. So bad I wanted a real family around her. No matter how drastic a change I made, I still wound up with the same family pattern I started with. There was no way out of the maze as long as I carried the same script inside that would attract a man exactly like my own father. And I'd react as a woman just as her mother did.

Here I went to the ends of the earth to marry an Arab, so drastically different from my own New York-born Jewish parents. And the Arab starts beating me, talking to me without respect-just like Meyer related to Tsipke.

Before I knew it I had an eighteen month-old daughter in the playpen and had already brought home a newborn son. "We're sending the kids to Syria," Ahmed insisted.

I was too weak to resist, but change had to come. This time it was inevitable. Instead of leaving him without even the shirt on her back, I developed agoraphobia. Afraid of separation, I built a prison around myself within the walls of my apartment. I was young, married, and still did not achieve my goal of living in my own private house rather than in a rented residence.

Agoraphobia and panic disorder took away my choices. I had realized now that I'd inherited the anxiety genes. There was no way I could step out of my home to leave, no way to cross the threshold by the time my son was six months old. At least those who couldn't walk push themselves in wheelchair. I could walk and still desperately yearned to be pushed in a wheelchair, to be taken care of. Someone had to care, but there was no one to care but me and a higher power if I could tap into it.

I withdrew to the house. I was in a sense married to my house in order to keep the family together. I held onto the home so dearly that I couldn't even get to the mailbox. Besides, loose dogs, big German Shepherds ran around the neighborhood biting anyone who wasn't in a car. That served to keep me locked inside the home where it wasn't so safe as I imagined. Think of agoraphobia, and think of loose dogs on top of it. There's no place like home.

◆   ◆   ◆

12

Spring 1967, Brooklyn, New York, Meyer's Apartment

I lived in Washington at the time with my children age two and six months, and was housebound with agoraphobia, so I and didn't see what happened, but mom told me that Samintov at 32, had been married to Benjamin for twelve years now. The Jewish mother of two descended the basement steps to put her laundry in Meyer's washing machine that he kept in the cellar. She was singing as she carried her family's wash down the darkened staircase.

Samintov and Benjamin rented an apartment in Meyer's four-family house. However, business was bad and Benjamin hadn't paid his 73-year old father rent in a long time. Meyer's brain damage problems were causing his extremely violent episodes to increase. Samintov wore her Israeli caftan that morning. Samintov switched on the red light in the basement that doubled as Benjamin's photo lab and walked across the cement floor past the dusty coal bins.

Suddenly Meyer jumped out of the darkness of the coal bin as Samintov began to load her laundry into the machine. Samintov jumped back as she saw a glimpse of Meyer's face under the red light.

He wielded his ax above his head and took a swing at Samintov * (name changed for privacy). As mom saw her looking up into dad's angry face. Mom said that she saw the mean swing in his arm just before he hit my brother's wife once at the back of her head and once on the side of her chin.

Samintov was able to scramble to her feet and crawl back up the cellar steps with Meyer slowly stalking her, yelling at her. "Why did you marry my son and ruin his life? You and your mother are nothing but troublemakers!"

Samintov made it to the top of the stairs. I pulled open the basement door. Light filtered through, blinding her. She limped through the tiled four plex hallway and out onto the stoops beside the small garden in front of the house before tumbling onto the sidewalk. Samintov's leg twitched like a freshly axed chicken.

"Heads will roll. I tell you heads will roll." Meyer followed her onto the street ranting. "Just like heads rolled in World War One in Tours."

Meyer continued to swing his ax over his head and to come after her. She looked back at him and screamed for her mother who lived next door.

"You people haven't paid rent in years. I'm losing my house. You hear?" Meyer stood over her.

Samintov's mother, Mazeltov* (name changed for privacy), was sitting on her white stucco Brooklyn stoop talking with her own elderly mother, Ribca When Samintov began to scream for her mommy, Mazeltov rushed over and grappled with Meyer, whom she had called the troublemaker.

She pulled the ax handle out of the elderly man's grip. Then Mazeltov began to hit Meyer with the handle of the ax until her own mother came running over with a hammer and handed it to her. At that, she began to beat Meyer &bout the head with her own hammer.

Neighbors flocked and pulled Mazeltov off of Meyer, but only after she covered his face with hammer blows.

"What did you do to my daughter? Why'd you cut my daughter? Mazeltov shouted.

"You 're daughter will be all right," a neighbor man assured her.

"Sit down, the police are coming."

Samintov's leg was still twitching as she lay on the sidewalk. Someone threw a blanket over her until the ambulance and the police arrived.

The neighbor led Mazeltov to the stoop. She sat and cried while the neighbors held a handkerchief to the back of Samintov's head and dabbed at her chin until she could get stitched up.

"The cuts don't look to bad. She'll always have a scar, though," the neighbor man told Mazeltov.

No one noticed the black and blue hammer marks on Meyer's face. He was still muttering, "Heads will roll! How dare you use my washing machine?"

Mazeltov ran forward and bent over him as the police ambulance paramedics placed him on the stretcher.

"What have you done to my daughter?"

"You scum of in-laws, put me in the poorhouse will you?"

"I hope you die for cutting my beautiful daughter's face."

The door of the police ambulance closed with a loud thud. Neighbors crowded around Samintov holding a handkerchief to the back of her head and her chin as the medics helped her onto a stretcher in the second ambulance.

Samintov moaned for her mother, and Mazeltov climbed in with her along with Mazeltov's elderly mother. The three generations of women crowded into the ambulance together.

"You were right, mommy. I shouldn't have married into that crazy cold fish family." Samintov sobbed loudly as the ambulance drove away.

A week later Samintov was scarred, but well enough again to resume her housewife duties back with her husband, Benjamin, the lawyer who paid all her bills. Her thirteen year-old daughter and eleven year old son were silent.

But Meyer's prostate gland swelled up on him again in the jail hospital. They operated on him again his will and he died the next day of fright fighting against the operation.

◆   ◆   ◆

13

The Same Day in May, 1967 in Ahmed's California Restaurant

I was slicing tomatoes. At the age of 25, I had a two-year old and a six-month old (a part-time babysitter and intermittent agoraphobia). I worked part-time as the cook in spite of my Master's degree in creative writing and in "the fine arts." By now, all I wanted to be was a creative director in an in-house ad agency and boss of my own creativity.

Instead I received phone calls from some woman who saw my paintings of mountain village life in ancient times hanging in my husband's restaurant and screamed, "I thought you could do better than that." She banged the phone shut. Why couldn't they learn that what they thought of my paintings was their own business, not mine? Praise I'll take anytime from anyone. I've earned it by now.

Finally, I got to do creative expression work after earning a masters degree in the creative arts and fiction writing. I cooked all the Middle Eastern food at Ahmed's restaurant and nightclub, Baal-Loves-and-Loses-Ashearah in California.

Sliced tomatoes flew into the dish. Hoda, the bellydancer at my husband's restaurant, a secondary school dropout with a Pakistani dad and Dutch mom now stood over me, supervising and criticizing when Ahmed had to help wait on the tables and play host. She was a decade older than I, more beautiful with long, black hair, blue eyes, olive skin, 36 DD cups, a tiny waist and big hips.

I stood next to her as she controlled and supervised my work. Me, 34 AA cups, waist and hips the same 35 inches, short legged, long-nose, scar faced, and … I shouldn't have to go through these comparisons. What did I have that I could sell? An IQ over 135, a Masters degree in English/Creative Writing, and a talent for both writing and art.

Why did she end up supervising me? I was divorced, unpaid, working for tips, and still living at home, dependent on my husband as an alternative to homelessness. He would soon kick me out into the street with twenty-eight cents to my name and no living relatives or friends to help me. I'd soon get the chance to swim, to make it on my own with agoraphobia and panic disorder.

Hoda, my husband's mistress had left strands of her long, black hair in my bed. She lived the earlier part of her life in Germany and the Netherlands and spoke with a thick, low-voiced Germanic accent. Ahmed stood in a corner talking softly to his mistress.

He kissed Hoda on her pierced, gem-stoned navel for good luck and touched the undersides of her bejeweled breasts. Hoda accidentally knocked a circle of pita bread from the counter top. Ahmed snatched the bread from the floor, kissed it and ate it, piece by piece.

"Bread is the symbol for life."

He raked his eyes over Hoda's metallic gold fabric costume as the band faded into nuances of oriental delight.

Beyond the double doors of the restaurant kitchen where I put in time, a magic world took center stage. There was a round platform where the oud-player stood, a place for the violinist and a pink light on the clarinetist. Sometimes Theodakis* (name changed for privacy), the Greek, from Alexandria, Virginia, came in to play his bouzouki. And Hoda twisted her grief through the sieve of a flute.

Between dance performances, there was the roar of rhumba drums covered with hairy hide. Then Hoda would rush out and coil so that the candles trembled.

Ahmed was dressed in a Tuxedo, his hair slicked back like a wet beaver. Now that Hoda had to get ready to dance, Ahmed walked over to I to peer over her shoulder. I had cut all the tomatoes in quarters.

"I distinctly told you I wanted fifths."

"I'll cut them my own way. Who's the cook around here, anyway?" I shot back, holding in her jealousy of Hoda.

"Are you sassing' me again?" Ahmed wheezed in his clipped, Arabic accent.

"They're going to get cut the way they look prettiest."

I thought-he prefers a mistress who spends her spare time sewing historical ethnic costumes for six-inch dolls.

"Why don't you ever listen?" Hoda flushed. "Quarter slices take up the whole plate."

"I don't take orders from my husband's whore."

"You nasty little bitch," Hoda grunted. "Get out of this restaurant."

"No! I've invested four thousand dollars of my insurance money in this place. It was my idea to start this restaurant."

They didn't know I had set up a tape recorder in a secret place and recorded all their conversation when they were alone. Later, I played it back many times to confirm my hunches about what went on between these lovers when they talked about me behind my back. I saved it for many years. Then I threw the tapes into a dumpster long ago when I had once dreamed that someday I would run up a pittance into glory in the stock market in my middle age based on my own researched picks. No such luck. Still penniless and one door knob away from being homeless. But I won't budge. I'm at home, and I won't venture out. It's so safe inside. Yeah, sure.

"Get the hell outta here!" Ahmed was a pool of anger.

He lifted I by the back of her blouse collar and threw her bodily out the kitchen back door into the alley where I fell against two garbage cans.

I promptly walked back into the restaurant, wanting a relationship so badly that I was willing to fight for it.

"I got my head smashed in while I was feeding my baby in the ear he was test driving and wrecked. All my insurance money that came for the masked epilepsy I have now for the rest of my life went into this restaurant. You didn't know that, did you, Hoda?"

"Why are you telling me all this?" Hoda was fixing her lipstick in her compact mirror.

"Now you're gonna get it," Ahmed ranted.

Instead of running, I waited, waited for an answer to come charging down on a white horse instead of going out and digging it up for herself.

Ahmed picked up the carving knife and ran after I. I bolted out the kitchen door and ran down the dark alley.

"Damn you," I screamed back as I ran. "I just came back for my purse. My keys are in it."

"I don't give second chances," Ahmed yelled.

He chased his wife, running more than a block down the neon-sign lighted street. He waved the knife over his head. I rounded the corner and disappeared into the night. Ahmed returned to his restaurant and calmly began to re-slice the quartered tomatoes into fifths.

"Did she go straight home?" Hoda asked.

"I don't know. She said her keys were in her purse."

"It's over there on the counter."

"I try to control her," Ahmed commanded. "But she's not obedient anymore."

"What about that psychiatrist that comes in here everyday for lunch?"

"He gave me his most expensive oriental carpets to store," Ahmed confessed.

"Maybe he'll testify for you so you can get custody of the kids."

"I know he will."

"Have you told I that the kids are going to live permanently with your mother in Syria after the divorce?"

"No. Not until she signs the quitclaim deed on the house and restaurant-and I sell them."

"Why would she willingly sign a quitclaim deed?"

"I told her the divorce was cancelled-that we were moving to Beverly Hills."

"How can that woman be so selfish?" Hoda adjusted her faux-pearls. "I'd kill anyone who tried to take my children away from me."

"She's riddled with panic disorder. No way can she support herself, let alone children."

"She gets dizzy just sitting at a restaurant table."

"If I divorce her now, she'll sign anything just so I deliver groceries to her door."

Ahmed popped a grape in his mouth. "There's no way she can step outside unless I drive her to the restaurant and leave her in the back where she won't have to talk to people."

He embraced Hoda and slipped his hand under her belt. "The little Jew Gypsy bastard's afraid to even talk on the phone. You know my psychiatrist friend?"

Ahmed shook his head. "He told me he diagnosed her as borderline paranoid."

"How can she just leave her children like that?"

The music echoed. Whirling dervishes spun like tops until they were hypnotized. The thumping grew louder, men yelled "Wah, wah, yalla, yells ay...." The pitch grew intense as the music faded ... into wailing nuances of Oriental delight. The audience ate up the act.

Then Hoda was on, under a beam of violet light. The rhythm pumped. An Irish whistle in E flat piped out the shrill music of ancient Egyptian wheat fields. The ceiling of the restaurant was blackened and lighted with stars like a planetarium dome.

A singer crooned the poem I had written years ago, and they used for free: "From her ruby navel poems contract."

Hoda snapped her gold whip, dressed like Isis, the ancient Egyptian goddess. Gold Egyptian tunic, fake leopard skin down her back, and the Isis headdress.

Twangs of the oud explored hot bubbles of lava. Hoda could go from pure Nesselrode to the burning passion of flamenco in Zamba Mora style in seconds, then to the world beat of Maghrebi Magham Seegah. Her Turkish finger zills clacked in time with the hand-clapping, feet thumping, the oud, the pipes, the dumbeka, tar, tom-tom, castanets of wooden spoons, the whirling dervishes on the circular stage.

Down Hoda's sallow breasts burst blue-black beaded braids, innocent as Eden to the audience. Each man in the audience viewed the other with mistrust. She did a back bend-applause. For a grand finale, Hoda ripped her skirt to show how she was cleft.

My flight for survival pushed down any symptom of agoraphobia or panic disorder for the moment. I hailed a taxi and ran to my next-door neighbor's house.

It was just like when she was pregnant-the anxiety attacks, the panic would disappear, only to return again full-blown when the baby was a week old.

The attack would be the only way she got touched. Battering was caressing. Being scared to death was feeling existence, having personal space of one's own, being recognized.

Only through pain could she act instead of react to him. Slowly the agoraphobia was worsening each time it came back. She dreaded having to look for a job, having to take the bus. Learning to drive, like flying, was out of the question.

My home grew on my skin. My fantasies were of having a loving husband and a big house in Beverly Hills with a pool and being a Jewish American princess with type AB+ Himalayan blood, nomadic as a Sumerian on the Silk Route to Rajasthan, yet Jewish as a Litvak from Grodno at a Coney Island Knish Stand.

Without husband and family, I, he balabusta, the great Shakespeare-reading homemaker, was separating from my self. And separation was unbearable. Yet I had trapped myself at home-his home, not ours, in the process of trying to cling to my last crumb of family solidarity. All I wanted was to dissolve boundaries between family members and myself. A twisted crumb is better than nothing at all.

◆   ◆   ◆

14

State Fair Parking Lot, Summer Of 1969

You'd go to any extreme to be the center of attention, even marry someone like me, just to have material for your novel or screenplay. So you can get rich?" Ahmed babbled to me as he parked the car.

The neighbor lady paid the taxi bill, since all Ahmed paid me was two quarters a day for ice cream for the kids. He brought home all the food from his restaurant.

I spent the night sleeping on my neighbor's sofa. Ahmed's two brothers lived with him and watched the children when I was in the restaurant.

Ahmed cooled down by the morning after spending the night with Hoda. By noon, almost everything was back to the same routine. But he never allowed me to set foot in his restaurant again.

The more Ahmed chased me with a carving knife, the more often he put his .38 against my head, or spit in my face and called me a "dirty Jew," the more physically well I felt.

It was only when he was charming to me or kind that my agoraphobia and panic attacks returned or that I had vertigo spells or migraines and went into convulsions of hyperventilation syndrome. Each time I fell into a sick complaint, he'd take off his shoe and whack me over the head.

I would provoke him. He'd attack and hurt me. I'd run for life and in the running process itself, I would feel alive with a sense of well-being, an adrenaline rush that would suppress the panic and anxiety that would well up when all was stagnant and routine calm.

Now 28, I pulled myself from the station wagon, dragging my four-year old daughter and two-and-a-half-year old son. I tried to walk a few paces, pushing the boy's stroller ahead of me.

I panicked at the idea of walking the stretch of parking lot. I turned to Ahmed, fearfully clutching at his middle in an attempt to get back a futile hug.

I was starving for skin contact. "I can't walk, I told you. I can't walk outside the house. Where's a wheelchair? Get me a wheelchair!"

"Goddammit! Walk, you whore! I said walk"

Ahmed slapped me in the face until his knuckles bled.

"Wheelchair! I want a wheelchair!"

"You're not a damn cripple! I didn't marry a crazy woman. You'd better walk, I tell you. I'm not going to push you in a wheelchair. Don't start that stuff with me again."

"Don't you ever call people with disabilities cripples," I scowled over my shoulder. "You don't know how badly I want to see the Del Mar Fair. I prayed for anything just to get out of the house after all these years. I can't walk," I sobbed, whining.

"Either you walk or you get the hell outta here!"

"I can't. I can't. Push me in the wheelchair, love me, nurture me, care about me. Be my mommy, my family. Love me."

"I'll kill you!"

"I demand to be pushed and to be cared for like a wife." I now ran before his fist again lashed out.

"You can go back alone, you whore." He sounded like daddy. People were staring and Ahmed didn't want anyone who might be a potential customer to see him lose his charm. He, exactly like husband number two, cared what the neighbors heard more than he cared to plan a time just for talking with me. The more he withdrew, the more verbal I became.

Husband one or two, it was the same.... withdrawal, uncaring.... me more verbal, asking for a relationship, begging to get closer through talking.... he becoming violent, putting hands around my throat ... when I asked him to respect me, to show less contempt.

Husband number one in 1970 hustled "his" children away from me and carried them tenderly back into his car. Ahmed sped away leaving a trail of dust for me to eat.

"Hey you didn't give me any money," I shouted to the empty air as the car disappeared.

A female security guard drove by, and I signaled her attention. "My husband and kids drove away without me, and I haven't a dime to get back home. Can you help?"

"Hop in."

"I'm sorry. I'm having another postpartum panic attack. My legs just turned to rubber. There's no way I can walk anywhere with this agoraphobia, probably caused by loss, grief, and a drop in hormones after childbirth causing this chronic anxiety in someone like me-genetically prone to get this panic disorder." My whole body shook with too much insulin and adrenaline. It subsided when I ate something.

"We'll call Traveler's Aide. You got a long way back to Hollywood. How do you know he won't turn back for you?"

"He won't. He's got the kids with him."

"My boss expects me to make everyone feel good."

"This was my first excursion out of the house in years. Agoraphobia with panic disorder, you know."

"Oh, the housewife's disease."

"And Mr. Take Away Man. He just wanted my American citizenship."

"Sounds like my own ex-husband ... the shortage. What you need is a good lawyer. "Sure. And who pays?" "Your husband." "He'd shoot me first." "Leave. Change your name. Get a new identity." "Oh, no-agoraphobia. It's genetic-a chemical imbalance.

The metabolism of the right brain goes at twice the speed as the left hemisphere. I could have been married to the President and I'd still get it worse after every childbirth, operation or heavy job stress."

◆   ◆   ◆

15

A Posh Hollywood Hotel, New Year's Eve 1969

A live band was playing the most romantic of music. The Hawaiian luau at fifteen dollars a person was something that I had saved up for a long time. She had received a fat check for the sale of her story to Saturday Review and was going to spend it on food and music.

Patrons waited in a long line for the oriental buffet. Couples danced on the wooden floor. The chandeliers pulsated. In a corner the Christmas tree was still up, decorated with love.

Ahmed and I ate together for the first time in months. He had always dined with his brothers in the restaurant or with Hoda, but never with me. The last time he ate with me he ended up throwing a vase in my head. With Hoda, he made love to her, and she confided in a customer that he was the worse lover she had. The customer, a friend of my then husband's brother told me that. So I don't know whether she made it up or Hoda really told her that.

Why does it feel good when you hear that your ex-husband is a selfish lover to the mistress for whom he left you? If he were a good lover, would it make any difference? No. You'll never have fun with him again anyway. So it's not important. Why do women talk to one another that way when they know you're newly divorced? Another woman said to me "I bet you just laid there and did nothing." I told her, "What difference does it make now?" See how often strangers will tell you what you already know about your appearance, attitudes, or your ex-husband?

The band played Auld Lang Syne, but Ahmed scowled with confusion. He wasn't going to let I move him to sentiment.

I thought about Christmas Eve. He had taken Hoda to a nightclub and brought home a bag of peanut shells for I to take down to the garbage cans.

A quarter to midnight. everybody was touching, dancing. Ahmed stared coldly across the table at I. "You don't need a lawyer of your own. My attorney will refer you to his attorney friend for a token seventy five dollars to keep it legal."

I sighed and crushed my napkin. "Why are you sending my babies to Syria?

"I want my mother to raise them as Muslims. Don't you dare tell that lawyer anything other than that you're giving up custody to me because you're in bad health."

"Why won't you answer my question?" I wept.

"It's too expensive to raise babies here. Besides, they'd only grow up to be Hollywood drug addicts or tramps, like all American kids."

"But you told me that if I signed the house over to you that you'd cancel the divorce. You said you needed the money for your restaurant liquor license."

Ahmed rose and put on his jacket. "Listen, I want a divorce. You're a stone around my neck. I want to be free."

"I don't know any man more free than you. Don't take my babies."

"You're too crazy to have babies."

"You can't take both of them. Let me have just one. Please don't leave me. I'll give you my parent's four-family house that my brother took away from me when they died."

"Shut up! I'm not separating my kids."

Twelve midnight cracked open the music. The band went wild playing nostalgia from the twenties. And the balloons and confetti flew around the ballroom.

Couples kissed and hugged and merged into one happy moment of celebration. I wiped the tears from my cheeks before anyone noticed how I trembled. I was unable to look Ahmed in the eye. Slowly I raised my head and looked around miserably at the frenzied couples hopping to the 1926 Charleston. Then the 1963 twist came on-sheer nostalgia now. Couples circled on the ballroom floor, laughing out loud. The drunks sprawled across their chairs.

"I paid for both of our dinners, Ahmed ... paid so we could be together again." He looked down at his shoes. "It's after twelve," he said. "I have to get back to close up my restaurant-see whether it's crowded."

"I won't go to that empty house alone. I want my justice." I gathered her jacket and purse.

Ahmed gave her the barber's itch. He pulled that little wisp of hair at the nape of my neck that gave me a terrific sting.

"Mi vida." Maybe I should have spoken in Arabic instead of Spanish. Could anything be said to make an impact? How does an INFP on the MBTI (Myers-Briggs Personality Type Indicator ®) talk to an ESTJ first husband, let alone an

ISFJ second husband? I knew a few words in a lot of languages, always wondering when I could use the phrases.

Could I use personality preference letter abbreviations as I would use foreign phrases? My husband dropped out of secondary school in Syria and went to Germany to work as a machinist at age 17. He wouldn't know what I was talking about. Or would he? He knew the power of silence. That's why he was clever as an immigrant businessman full of potential. Yet he ended up penniless. If only he didn't chase me with a carving knife or try to loop a thin wire around my neck to strangle me. I outran him. Why couldn't he simply say, let's divorce and divide the community property.

No, he couldn't use words. All he could do was to take me on a two-day vacation while he quietly took the children out of the country and all the money in our joint bank account. He placed them to be raised by his mother and six brothers in Syria. Fifteen years passed before I saw them again as devout Muslim college students whose greatest fear was the Arab community finding out my great grand daddy was a learned rabbi. When my children had children, their greatest fear was that their children would find out.

Find out what, that I'm a secular American who goes to meetings of the Freethinkers clubs just to listen to lectures on parallel universes? Or that I read Darwin? Or that I celebrate the Federal holidays by looking at decorative trees in shopping malls? Or enjoy a talk on new-age healing with harp music at an interfaith hall? Or paint Tibetan-style mandalas for relaxation?

"If you open your mouth to anyone, you'll be dead in twenty-four hours," he warned me.

"I called my brother for help yesterday. His wife answered the phone. I told her I wanted to take the kids back to New York, to come home again. You know what she said? She told me to drop dead or go on welfare."

"If you want money, go out and earn it like everybody else, you human garbage."

"For ver tu care morena, al Dio dare mi alma!"

I turned away because he spit in my face.

But Ahmed had turned and didn't mind me turning my head to avoid his spit. I heard only Sicilians spit at you when they're angry. No, lots of Mediterranean cultures spit. Now I saw the full brunt of his anger once more. He'd pay attention only to my actions, not my reactions.

"Are you coming home? I said I have to get back to the restaurant!"

Now he'd fired me up. "Back to your whore, Hoda? You hire a pitiful forty-year-old bellydancer more than ten years older than I am and you break up the family. For her you steal my babies and try to kill me, for a tramp with a grown daughter."

"You're gonna get it later tonight, you flat-cheated, four-eyed dirty Jew Gypsy bitch!"

He slapped his hand against his belt and his thigh and punched his fist into his palm.

The hotel ballroom took on the tense and tedious gray tones of a madhouse. "You filed for divorce papers just two days after you became an American citizen. Then you flew to New York and borrowed a thousand dollars from my brother."

"Go to hell," Ahmed belched.

He stormed out, shoving the dancing couples out of his way. She yelled across the ballroom floor at him as he passed through the doorway. "My sister-in-law thinks I'll ask my brother for support money. Hoda told me you're the worst lover she's ever had. Are you gay?"

Ahmed pivoted. "What did you call me?" There was fire in his jade green eyes. He came over and grabbed her on the dance floor, shaking her violently. He threw her to the floor and kicked her in the kidneys. I screamed, but he clenched his hands over her lips.

"Wife batterer!" She moaned, lost among the dancing feet and drowned out by the magic brass. The crowd was hell bent on yelling its own celebration. I pulled her arm out of Ahmed's grip and ran to the door, screaming.

"Lower your voice! Don't you hear me?" Ahmed followed her out of the hotel. "I said can you lower your voice? I'll stifle that anger. Just wait 'till I get you alone at home tonight, you whore." That's what my father always called me. Neither had reason to. Why would they call a faithful woman who remained a virgin on her wedding night such a name, or a studious girl who hid behind thick glasses and astronomy books such a term? What did it do for them?

◆   ◆   ◆

16

Our Living Room New Years Eve 1969 at 2:00 A.M.

The radio played the instrumental version of "Ave Maria." I sat on the tweed sofa staring off into space. But Ahmed couldn't sit still. He paced back and forth, trapped as a caged lion, waving his .38 handgun at me. Finally, he pointed the gun against my head.

"You're not a Nazi. I trust you with my life," she whispered.

"Do you?" Ahmed squealed. "I want custody of my children. You're jailing me. Too damn dependent, you are. I'm divorcing you and sending the kids to my mom in Syria. You told your own mother you wished a doctor married you. Now you'll have your chance."

"What I told her when she was alive was that I gave up a doctor for you."

"You're nothing but a 'nobody.' Why would a doctor look at you?"

"To examine me when I pay him," I responded, timorously.

"Why would a lady doctor look at you? Would you want your daughter to marry a man exactly like you? "I sighed. I hope your daughter becomes a doctor or marries one that treats her kindly. If I didn't marry one, I hope my children will." It made me think that my mother said she wished I'd marry a doctor because she couldn't marry a doctor. And her dad went to medical school for a while, until he had to leave for America in a hurry around 1890 because of the pogroms in Europe. My daughter did marry a doctor who does treat her kindly.

My son became a doctor. Perhaps the grand daughters will become doctors as well as marry them, I thought. I have many grand daughters and grand sons. There's only one catch. I'm forbidden to tell them that my great grandparents were Jewish and from Poland. Why should it matter? They're Arabs. They go to Islamic schools. There's social stigma.

Do they know by now Arabs and Jews share some Middle Eastern genes and a language group. It didn't help the Hatfields and the McCoys, Scots-Irish families in America who may have shared similar genes. If sharing a common ancestor in the Middle East or West Asia can't make people be friends with one another, what can help people be closer and love one another? I thought this was my job to make peace at the family level. Emotionally, I arrived in peace and left in pieces. Now, there are celebration of life ceremonies at interfaith houses of worship. What else beckons me? Kaballah's secrets? Tell me more. I'm seeking a best friend who will not threaten my serenity and home.

"So I wasn't good enough for a Jewish American Princess-with a lawyer for a brother? My first husband chided."

"So I wasn't good enough for a rich Jewish doctor," I replied.

Ahmed pulled off the wedding ring on my skinny finger and spit on it.

I whined "You lied. You told me that your had a PhD in mechanical engineering. I married you because I wanted a professional man for a husband. You were a dropout from some high school, a machinist in a German factory for six years. You knew exactly what you wanted when you married me."

"So I'm not good enough for you?"

I'm a rich girl without money. I'm not a poor girl. But you-you lied every inch of the way."

"Fortune hunter!"

"For you I went to college almost six years?"

"And what have you got to show?"

"Class, taste, dignity! Books on art history."

"And I've got a quarter of a million dollars from the sale of my restaurant." Ahmed squeezed her cheeks together with two fingers until her mouth puckered.

"I'm divorcing you because you're a cold fish in bed." Ahmed watched my expression. "After two children, who'd want to look at you with your chicken flesh, stretched out belly and flat chest?"

"Am I that bad of a mother? Please, please don't break up the family. It's all I have left."

Ahmed removed his shoe and whacked her over the head. He spit in her face. Then he fondled his pistol. "You know what Hoda did on Christmas Eve? She sucked my cock twice."

"Go to hell, you bastard." I ran into the bedroom in tears. I suddenly realized that what I had left was myself, my self respect.

I wanted to make peace between Arabs and Jews starting at the family level. What if we all realized where came from—mama Africa, then India, the Gulf, and then the whole world sang and reflected every corner of it at different moods?

"I'll kill you. Sharmutter! Whore!" Ahmed flung the Turkish coffee pot at me. "If you give me any trouble."

"Don't take my babies. I can't break up the family. What else have I got, except myself and my ambition in a world where I'm really not wanted?"

Ahmed looked up at me wide-eyed. I had given him a new idea. He locked up his gun and phoned the police. "My wife is going to commit suicide." He was calm and cool on the phone. I'm divorcing my wife and she's threatened to take her own life. Please come quickly."

"What?" I paled. "You're calling the police to develop a record of suicide reports on me when you know I'd never do such a thing? You're doing this just to build a record so you'll get custody of the kids, you bastard!"

"I'm divorcing you." Ahmed repeated, still on the phone with the police. Gamal * (name changed for privacy)—Ahmed's brother walked into the house. He laughed for no reason, viewing the arguing couple.

"Your ulcers acting up again?" Ahmed called to his younger brother.

Ahmed motioned for his brother's help. The two men exchanged conversation in Arabic. Suddenly Gamal and Ahmed grabbed me and dragged me across the living room floor. Gamal was laughing and speaking loudly in Arabic. I was bare-foot, wearing my flimsy negligee. My hair flowed to my waist and he made sure he pulled it.

They dragged me into the bathroom and pushed my face close to the mirror. Ahmed whipped out a razor blade from his shaving kit and held it against my wrist as Gamal laughed crazily, not interfering with his brother's taming of his wife.

"I can kill you, if I want to. You know that. And I can tell the police it was just one more suicide attempt." Ahmed rubbed the razor back and forth against her wrists, not making any marks. Then he put it down and slapped her until her mouth bled. Ahmed bent her head down into the toilet.

"See the crap stains you left unscrubbed? You'd better clean this house, you lazy asshole ... I've got to sell it." He pushed her head into the bowl and flushed. Then he pulled mer out as I coughed and choked on the swirling water.

I saw myself as a tiny woman hurled into the blackness of the night air as Ahmed's door slammed shut in my face. I banged on the door pleading to be let back in. But my cries went unanswered. Inside Ahmed phoned the police again. I pressed her ear against the window to hear the conversation.

"I want to report my wife is trying to kill herself. Hurry over here. My two babies are sleeping soundly in the bedroom, and I don't want my ex-wife back in here.

"Yes, I have the interlocutory decree of divorce in my pocket. No, she doesn't live here. This is my house. She said she had no place to stay, but Gypsies are like that, nomadic. They stay anyplace. Can you get her out of here pronto?" I hugged the walls of the small, stucco house. Then I sidled down the walkway to the neighbor.

"Gypsies? Where did that come from?" He was telling the police I was a Gypsy. He didn't even use the politically correct term, Romani or Rroma. He'd say anything to maintain custody of the children so he could send them to Syria as he did. And I never saw them again until they grew up and returned as adults demanding food and money for college, but forbidding me to say I had Jewish relatives.

Oh, in private, when they were grown they acknowledge it, spoke friendly about it, but hid my writings and forbid me from telling their children I was well, Jewish via my relatives. But I attended the Unitarian church most days and once a year went to the temple to light a candle for my great grandparents. I understand they fear social stigma from their Arab friends.

My grandchildren will never know that before their mom, their ancestors were Jewish at least for a thousand years in Europe if not longer. Where are we going? Quo Vadis? Can I be Christian, Jewish, Hindu, Buddhist, Muslim Humanist, Unitarian, and everything else and still feel the divine love?

Is there anything out there other than design? I'm into Ayurvedic medicine and philosophy. Where did I come from? Mother India? Where do I belong—ultimately? I have a need for a core identity, but I can't share it with relatives for all that's left are my children and grandchildren. Where do I belong? Who am I? These thoughts run like a river seeking an ocean that as the popular song reverberates, "will not refuse the river." And at age 27, Ava was my Australian friend who lived next door.

Ava was a British immigrant married to a Pima Indian. The light was still burning in Ava's living room. I peered through her window and watched Ava sitting on the sofa next to her husband. The middle-aged couple cuddled, snuggling up to each other. Their fireplace was ablaze, and the TV set was on.

I could hear the dance music on TV from the Times Square broadcast. She pounded on the door begging to be let in. A fine drizzle had started, and I shivered beneath her transparent negligee, My bare feet strained wet and caked with mud.

Ava jumped up as I pressed her face against the window. "What happened? Why are you here at this hour?" I ran in as soon as she opened her door. "I don't know where to go."

"We were just going to bed straightaway."

"He threw me out."

"Please let me sit here for a moment." She sat herself in Ava's rocking chair.

"He said he's divorcing me and taking the kids to dump on his mother in Syria. Don't believe him if he tells you I'm planning to commit suicide. Ahmed keeps calling the police and telling them I'm going to do it-just to build up a record. He needs a reason why he's entitled to custody."

"Why would your husband act crazy?"

"Don't you understand? He wants custody of the children. Building a record of suicide reports at the police station is easy. Every time they come over I get a light shined into my eyes and they look at my wrists and go away."

"A woman is nothing without a man." Ava poured her a cup of lukewarm tea that was standing on a small table. "A woman without a man is always in danger when she gets old. She'll be attacked on the street by grinning teenagers who hate her race."

I sighed. "A woman without a man can go to bed knowing she'll still be alive in the morning."

"I've got multiple sclerosis," Ava scowled. "Who'd take care of me if my husband left? There's nobody else."

"I'm not crazy, I tell you," I whined. "But my psychiatrist betrayed me. He played back to my husband the recorded tapes he made of our session-after he promised me our conversation would be confidential."

"Are you going to let him get away with that?" Jose, Ava's husband butted in.

"Who would believe me? The doctor is my husband's best customer and friend. He even stores the doctor's expensive rugs for him."

"How'd he set after he heard the tapes?" Ava brought out some leftover cake.

"Beat the hell outta me."

"You're just going to hand over your kids to him?"

"He told me to tell the lawyer my health was bad. Do you think he'd let me live one hour if he thought I'd run back home to New York with my kids?"

"His kids? It's your divorce. What about those stretch on your belly and those episiotomy scars?"

"I don't have money of my own. He took the money I earned from my freelance writing to magazines that I'd deposited in our joint bank account. When he changed the account or canceled it, I had no access to remove any money I earned. When you mix your income, the meager two hundred dollars I earned from the sale of an article, you lose any money you earned. He never let me have access to the joint bank account even though both our names were on it.

He put a gun in my head and warned me not to touch the account. I made a mistake depositing my earned money into our joint bank account."

"Grocery money?" Ava was grasping at anything.

"He brings all the food home from the restaurant or goes shopping. I can't step into a supermarket without getting a dizzy spell and panic attack. It's my agoraphobia."

"My goodness, look at you, I. You're a goner with that man." Jose left the room, disgusted.

"Don't you see? I can't ever open my mouth."

Ava saw the flashing lights and went to her window. "A police car stopped in front of your house."

"I told you he calls them every time we start to talk because he wants me out. He tells them I'm committing suicide each time. It's the only way he can get custody of the kids.

"Bull. You're signing away custody of the kids to him because you're really afraid he'll kill you."

"He beats me where it doesn't leave any marks, except inside my mouth. I can't leave my house without a panic attack. How can I support kids?"

"He sure hits below the belt when you're in the pits."

"Ahmed even forced me to sign a quitclaim deed to the house. He said he cancelled the divorce he started last year and he needed the money for his liquor license."

"And you believed a wife beater?"

"He said he canceled the divorce. Oh, your right! Is this what childbirth does to a woman's logic?"

"Babies can be crazy makers."

"Not with the right man."

"Even with the right man, Ava. Wouldn't it be great to wake up in the morning and know that you're still alive-that no one-man, relative, or jealous woman-would kill you while you slept?"

"Just walk away."

"Impossible. There are loose dogs in these dead-end streets. The neighbors just let their German shepherds roam free during the day when the streets are empty. I'm the only one who doesn't drive around here. The dogs attack me."

"Taxi?"

"To where? With no money? No friends? No living relatives to call on for help anymore?"

Ava ran her fingers through her shaggy blonde hair. "You're a love junkie, you are. You must thrive on natural highs, self-made panic attacks. Do you miss the action?"

"I want a caring family more than anything else in the world."

"You've got a prison for a home."

"I know. At the astrology convention years ago, someone looked at my chart and told me this. Mars in Aries in the seventh house of partnerships square Venus in Capricorn in the fourth house of home life and domesticity."

"That's nonsense superstition. Maybe you just don't want to do the dirty work to support yourself. We can't all be princesses."

"I've always felt I'm somebody special. That I was meant to be a princess. I'd rather be famous than loved."

Ava shook her head with impatience. "I've got to get to bed."

She locked the door as I hurried out. She waved to her and peered out of her window watching I walk back home in the rain. The police car was still parked in front of my house. "I'm okay," I whispered as the police officer shined a flashlight in her eyes looking for signs of drug use. "I'm a strict macrobiotic vegetarian." He looked at my tongue and turned my hands over to examine each wrist. As usual, they found no signs other than my high anxiety symptom complaints or hyper-ventilation syndrome, my asthma, or the shakes.

"Can you make her go?" Ahmed asked the police officer as I sat down on my own sofa. "It's my house," my husband insisted. Where's my house? I thought.

"Don't you have your own house to go to?"

"No. My husband sold it after he got me to sign a quitclaim deed when he convinced me he cancelled the divorce."

"But this is his house. You're divorced."

"Ahmed moved all my things in here when he sold my house. He bought this place for himself and his brothers because it's around the corner from his restaurant."

Ahmed pulled a piece of paper from his shirt pocket. "Here's my interlocutory decree of divorce."

The officer read the paper. "You need a lawyer, lady." I don't have a dime to my name."

"We did have a suicide attempt report."

"My husband just wants custody of the kids. That's why he called you. I never said a word to him or even thought of suicide. He makes up things to get custody of the children whom he's planning to send to his mom to be reared in Syria.

Won't anyone help me? I have no money and no place to go. My parents are dead, and I have no relatives or friends to turn to for help."

"Isn't there any way I can get this woman out of my house? My kids are asleep in there."

"I signed custody of the kids to him because I couldn't step out of the house to support them with this agoraphobia, panic attacks, and panic disorder. What if I change my mind and want my kids back? Every week he says he's canceling the divorce. Last week he said if I signed the house over to him, he'd cancel the divorce. I did so he could by a license for his restaurant. He promised he would cancel the divorce."

"I'll have her arrested for kidnapping." Ahmed snapped his fingers. He pulled out the divorce papers. No, he did not cancel the divorce. Why did I want to believe him? Why was I so afraid of finding a job and then quickly getting fired? Why did I cringe at the thought of having to walk out of my house? The agoraphobia, I decided created anxiety when I tried to walk to the mailbox.

The loose dogs would chase me, large German Shepherds from the neighbor down the block who worked all day. The dogs got out no matter how many times I sent letters. And then there were the loose pit bulls across the street, between me and the bus stop. I called so many times, but nothing happened.

The dogs ran loose for six years up and down the streets, between me and the bus to the freedom of seeking work. And then the babysitting fees. I had no money. If my husband found a baby sitter, it was always his mistress, the belly dancer. I had no choice in childcare. He ran the home as if he was the dictator of a foreign country, and he looked like a body double in face, coloring, and behavior of Saddam Hussein. In fact they both were born in the same year, 1937.

"But he's kidnapping my Jewish babies and taking them to his mother in Syria to be raised as Muslims."

"A father doesn't have any less rights to his kids or faith than a mother," the officer quipped. "But who you really need is a lawyer."

"I'm the one who spent hours in labor and then months recuperating from the hormonal change and episiotomy stitches and stretch marks and migraines."

"She can't work. She's crazy." Ahmed sneered. "I want her out of my house, away from my babies."

I began to hyperventilate. "He's not a good provider."

"All we can do is drive her to the rescue mission."

"Not with the bums and wings," I groaned.

"Look you two, it's New Years Eve. Can you let her stay just until morning?" The officer extended his hand to bargain with Ahmed, getting eye contact.

"You mean in America, a foreign man can just throw his wife into the streets at night and take away her kids just because she has no family to stand up for her?" I pleaded with the officer.

"Your brother hates you." Ahmed squinted.

"He's in the hospital dying of diabetes and his 350 pounds of overweight. His wife is going nuts thinking that I want him to give me money. That's why she hung up on me and told me to disappear. So I disappeared."

"Say, why don't you two kiss and make up. Everything will be okay in the morning," the second officer insisted.

My voice cracked. "He'll kill me if I try to stay in this house. My babies are in his bedroom and I'm locked out, always on the outside. Don't you understand? He's sending them to his mother in Syria-forever. A Jew can't roam all over Syria trying to take back her babies from their Muslim father. Can't you see I'm powerless?"

"She can stay until dawn, officer. I'm not going to touch her. Ahmed knew he had won.

"Pray he lets me live until morning. Last week he tried to strangle me with a wire. The week before he chased me with a knife. Tonight he and his brother dragged me into the bathroom and put a razor to my wrists. He makes up this story about suicide."

"She's under mental treatment with my psychiatrist."

"Disturbed? Hell, no I'm outraged. When a woman is outraged instead of hysterical, then, they call her crazy."

I began to weep quietly. "Did you hear him say his psychiatrist?"

"Now don't get hysterical, lady. We've got to be going." The officer patted her on the hand. "These domestic calls are the pits," The second officer said to his partner as they left. "He's not going to bother you. Just leave in the morning. You can go down to legal aid and fill out an application."

"Legal aid is for the poor. I'm still married to a rich man."

"The party is over, folks. Good night."." The officer finished his report and walked to his car.

"We don't drink. It's haram, forbidden," Ahmed shouted back, bubbling with his conquest as he quietly locked the door. Ahmed bolted himself in the bedroom with the kids.

I dressed and finally lied down on the sofa in my overcoat until daylight came. I saw that Ahmed had left his wallet on the coffee table. In a flash she cleaned out two fifty-dollar bills and change for bus fare.

Before anyone else in the house woke up, I had packed and sneaked out. For the first time since the birth of my daughter in 1965 and son in 1966 and the onset of agoraphobia/panic disorder, was I able to take a bus alone to the YWCA and get a cheap room. Never before in my life was I on my own and so utterly isolated.

As I child I didn't know where the boundaries between myself and my parents began or ended. Now, I missed the boundaries between my children and myself or my husband and the nest of family life.

Standing alone forced itself on me like a vortex when Saturn turned into Taurus in my eight and ninth houses of partner's money and foreign relationships and travel opposite my second house of money and emotions in Scorpio. In short, all my money, possessions, real estate, children, and relatives were swept away from me, and separation/divorce became real.

The lesson I had learned from all this vortex sweeping away was to take responsibility for sensible financial planning and to never count on children to be with you when you need a family most. Nobody is a security blanket for somebody else all the time. I become tired of magical thinking, tired of the power of astrology over me, bearing down to become stronger than a divine, loving God.

I needed kind solace. I'm tired of hearing fate and destiny predictions. I want to take control of my life and behavior. Enough surprises, enough of a vortex. When can I tap into a higher power that is eternally loving and gives me back control of the healing power with which I was born?

An inner voice kept nagging: You can't make it without a man to pay the bills. No one will hire you for long. Your health will fall apart. You'll always be fired for incompetence.

Resisting, I kept telling myself: I can support myself. I'm a college graduate with a master's degree in English, in creative writing. Someone out there will pay me, will allow me to survive Who will allow me, but myself?

When all else fails, when you have nothing to sell but yourself, you sell yourself. Not your body if only because it's ugly. You write a movie, a play, or a monologue about your life. You commercialize your memoirs and survive on the pittance until you take responsibility.

Another voice pounded in her solar plexus: No, no my body is too sensitive to stress. I'll fall apart and disappear. My self will disappear. The second battle I won. I made it to the "Y" in one piece and had my lightweight portable typewriter with me.

◆   ◆   ◆

17

December 22, 1971: My Furnished Room, Before Dawn

After Ahmed threw me out of his newest house. I took a furnished room four blocks from his restaurant. It was really a garage studio in back of a house.

Each time I would open the front door, I'd step right into the bathtub that was covered by a plywood board. There was an old fashioned bathroom sink next to the tub, a hotplate right above the sink, a toilet, all perched on a white lino-leum-over-cement-slab floor covered by a braided cotton throw rug.

The studio couch served as a bed. My old portable typewriter and a stack of K-Mart paper stood on a small writing table. The desk chair was draped with sweaters and stockings. A Mickey Mouse lamp stood on a particle board bureau drawer.

All for $75 dollars a month rent. Outside the window the rain was lashing against the leaky windows as the chill crept through the stucco building. The whole room was one oblong box, everything done in faded dark brown by the landlady. I added touches of her favorite color, coral. Ahmed had delivered her sewing machine to her, and I had spent Thanksgiving alone, sewing the white lace pillows and white on white quilt tops.

At five in the morning there was a knock on my door. She pushed herself out of the soft, mildewed mattress. Standing in the rain was Ahmed under a wide umbrella, wearing an Astrakhan cap and wool jacket with a Persian lamb collar. In front of him stood her five-year old daughter dressed in a bright red faux fur coat and hat. Holding little Sara's hand was David, her four-year old son all decked out in a suit and bow tie, carrying his little fire engine.

"We came to say goodbye," Ahmed smiled, squinting through half-shut lids. "The plane leaves in two hours."

"Are they going all by themselves?

"Sure," Ahmed boasted. "Their clothes are tagged. The stewardess will see that they get to the right city."

"Aren't you going to Syria with them?"

"No, what do you think I'm operating, a whorehouse? I've got a restaurant to run."

"Your mother will take care of them?" I asked.

"She's raised six boys. And look how I turned out."

Ahmed and the children walked in and sat down on the chair, the bed. "Sara, you look beautiful," I said.

"I've brought you the Dancerina doll you wanted for so long. Hi, there Davy. I got you the airplanes you wanted, the one from the toy store you used to be' me to buy."

I placed the toys in each of the children's arms and watched them dance and squeal with joy.

"Why did you have to go and buy them bulky toys like that for? How can I send them with those things on a plane?"

I looked askance at Ahmed. "You'll probably never allow them to see me again. I wanted them to remember me with something joyful."

"Next year I'll visit them or whenever I visit my mother again," Ahmed added.

"You mean you're dumping the kids on your mother to raise, but won't let me see them or visit me? And where are you going, to be free to travel the world and have your girlfriends? What am I supposed to do as a mother, since nobody is hiring me for a job to support myself?"

I looked up at the leaking ceiling, hugging myself. "I'll take any job so I can be financially independent. Why did you have to sell the house? There was only thirty-two hundred dollars of equity in it. My payments would have been only a hundred and fifty a month. Now you made me a homeless shopping bag lady now and in my old age."

"What do you need a house for? You're a single woman of thirty. You can travel now, go back to school, work, and find a husband."

"A house is my whole life," I sobbed. "How can I plan for my old age and retirement? Where will I work and how will I save money for the future, since no one is taking care of me and I have no more living relatives I know of, at least anyone who cares about me, and certainly nobody out here."

"You have a teaching job now."

"My classes in adult school closed because too few students registered. And how can I travel if I can't take a bus more than two miles because of the agoraphobia?"

Ahmed lighted a cigarette, running his fingers along the dust on top of my desk table. "Don't you ever clean this place? Boy, are you a crappy housekeeper." He shook his head and coughed up phlegm, spitting into the sink. I lived in a tiny converted garage in the back of a rich lady's home, a lady who never socialized with me, ever …

"Please don't smoke in my room. It's the only personal breathing space I have." I began to pace nervously. Then I hugged the children closer as they jumped wildly on the narrow convertible sofa mattress.

I coaxed them to settle down in my lap as they sat on the bed. Ahmed rocked back and forth sitting at my desk.

"Come and work for me in the restaurant. But I can't pay you. You'll have to work just for tips alone."

Twisting my hair didn't hold down the anxiety. "What I can't understand is why I gave you back the house after you offered it to me in the divorce papers! You promised you'd cancel the divorce if I gave you the house back even after you signed it over to me in the divorce papers. Then you asked me to sign a quit-claim deed.

Why did I believe you after you beat me and spit in my face? What's wrong with my logic? Your restaurant partner had the nerve to call me up and ask me to give you the house-said you needed it for your liquor license. I mean after the divorce?"

For a moment what flashed in my mind was who wrote the Bible and who checked for inconsistencies? There were the Ten Commandments with "Thou shalt not kill," and there was Exodus 35:2, obliging people of the book to strike down those working on Shabbat, the Sabbath. And Leviticus 11:10 chided followers not to eat shellfish and Leviticus 19:27 forbidding men of the people not to cut their hair. So either the proofreader checking the Bible for inconsistencies missed a few, or the Bible was written by humans with all the errors humans make, and no one checked for inconsistencies before copying the scroll.

How could you kill those who worked on the Sabbath but obey one of the Ten Commandments not to kill? And along came Jesus in the New Testament saying Love One Another. So maybe I needed to keep on reading all the Bibles of the world looking for those good books that had no violence. Isn't love all there is? I know because I heard it from the mouth of a Charlie Manson follower speak the lines in the movie Helter Skelter. The whole order of control was rather controlling. And here I was trapped in the prison of my own agoraphobia with another wife-beater, and the family was leaving in pieces having had arrived in peace.

The family was breaking up. My children were being shipped to Syria, and nobody would help me if I couldn't come up with five hundred dollars to pay a lawyer. I couldn't step out of the house or get beyond the mailbox. No man chained me in the house. Agoraphobia kept me housebound. As if the bonds were made of anxiety like fine lace, and they were inside.

Ahmed combed his hair in the mirror above the desk. "We've got to go now. Davy, kiss your mother goodbye."

"But why was I stupid enough to believe you and hand my house over to you just because you said the divorce was canceled?"

Ahmed waved I away with the back of his hand. "Hurry it up, Sara. Use the toilet."

"I guess it's time to start a new life, but too late for a new family. I could never go through another pregnancy again with all that vertigo and panic attacks afterward."

Sara and Ahmed looked up at I. "Gee I hate kids," she said to them. "But not you. How can I love you when your old man is taking you away?"

"You little bitch, Jewish whore." Ahmed murmured as he spat. "Dirty Jewish scum."

"Wow, a lot of names for a man to call his wife in front of the preschool-age children," I sighed. "And especially when you just took all the money from the joint bank account and borrowed thousands from my brother, then filed for divorce the day after. I noticed you filed only days after you received your citizenship papers.

"Your father has total control," I told my preschool children. "How can you love something that is totally controlled by the man who wants to see you destroyed? I know you will reject me because I am powerless now and wiped out by this vortex." I didn't want the children to hear all this. I spent my own childhood listening to my mother complaining bitterly about my father's neglect and beatings.

Ahmed opened the door letting the wind and rain rush in. "Don't you want to get a last look at your kids?"

"There'll be no part of me left in you soon, except at the molecular level. You'll be a Jew in your unconscious dream, always rejecting that part of yourself that's me. I bet he'll tell you I gave you two up, not that he took you from me with a gun at my head."

"See?" Ahmed panted. "The doctor told me you're borderline paranoid."

"Sure. My husband turns on the gas jets while I'm asleep and three months pregnant and later tries to strangle me with a thin wire, chases me a block with a carving knife, and puts a weapon in my head warning me not to fight for custody, and you think I'm borderline paranoid?"

"Paranoid," he repeated, licking his lips.

"Seems that way only around you, buster." I tossed on my heavy flannel robe. "My chronic anxiety neurosis is from stress. Maybe I have post traumatic stress anxiety from all those attack on me in the subway by black men who hate me because I'm white. And maybe you can add that to almost getting strangled and raped, plus having a father who chases me with a hammer and beats my mom, or a brother whose temper is threatening, or a husband who beats me—plus getting beaten in a train for looking like one ethnic group. It all adds up. Name one person who ever gave me a hug and meant it without crushing my ribs."

I tired of the thought that the auto accident when he drove and I sat in the back at age 25 had smashed in the left side of my head and left me with on-and-off vertigo for the rest of my days that helped to keep my agoraphobia and fears, my post traumatic stress disorder going. And later the painful, red swollen gums persisted into old age. I didn't understand why the husbands that I married had been Mr. Take-Away-Men, men that forbid me to receive the warmth, gentle touch, and smiling eyes basic to thriving at an infantile level.

"Why did you pose as an Arab housewife all these years—in a Jewish neighborhood of Brooklyn?"

"Because it was more challenging than posing as an Italian housewife in little Italy married to the Italian boy next door who pissed on me when I was a kid. I just wanted to see how far I'd have to travel in core identity to find kindness, hugs, and love. I still was looking for a daddy who would say you're too good for that when I misbehaved instead of chasing me for blocks waving a hammer over my head. I can't outrun men any more. I'm tired, and I have a lot of love to give, if I can conquer anxiety."

"It will stay with you because you were born with anxiety."

"What Jew in her right mind wouldn't feel paranoid around a family of Arabs who keep taking from her and turning on the gas jets when she's asleep?"

"Me? I've offered you a chance to work in the restaurant for tips. What ex-husband would still do that?"

I hugged and kissed the children. "Sara, promise mommy you'll be a doctor. Davy, study your mathematics and do something important so people will respect you."

"What are you saying to them?" Ahmed laughed.

"Because I always wanted to get a doctorate degree in something exciting and I never could save enough money or get good enough marks in something financial, so I have this master's degree in English with a writing emphasis. Am I employable with this, employable enough to support myself without a husband in old age? And math, well, I failed every math course I ever attempted. I want them to make of themselves so much more than I did."

"You're not dumb."

"Ahmed, I'm just an average, ordinary girl, an overachiever. I'm persistent and determined, and I never quit anything I like to do. It's just that I'm a failure because I could never pass fifth grade math-like my mom. The world doesn't value anything I do perform well, it demands I pass math or fail. So I failed."

"My kids are smart," Ahmed said. "I want them to make of themselves so much more than I did."

"They will."

Ahmed grabbed me by the shoulders and shook me violently. "Look at you. A Master's degree in fiction writing and a bachelor's degree in screenwriting. Why the hell do you have to play the martyr to write? What are you, Jesus Christ? I dropped out of school at fifteen. When I sell my restaurant next year, I'll take back a quarter of a million with me to Syria."

"You've lifted yourself up by my bootstraps." I buttoned up the children's coats. "When I met you I had a full-time job checking out books in the New York Public Library. Four nights a week I went to the university and persisted for six years with a B-plus average until I earned my two degrees. How did 1 fall so far after marriage and motherhood?"

"You're absolutely nuts."

"That's the only behavior you repeat, Ahmed, to call me crazy. But I have many alternatives in my ego-strength. Do hormones train a mother to be so dependent?"

"Maybe your nursing milk ended up in your brain."

I pointed my index finger at myself. "Why did this overeducated, dedicated career woman fall so far after marriage, Ahmed?"

"You never obeyed me!"

"Feel a little out of control? What nun's vows did I ever take to obey? Right after the birth of each baby, when you wanted to punch your fist right through my navel, I knew then that I shouldn't have had children. You weren't support-ing me through the recovery period. Do you know what lack of sleep does to a new mother? No night nanny for the first three months like Jewish American Princesses get if they demand it."

"Didn't you always dream of being that J.A.P.? You can have that career now."

"Career? I want a husband to support me and pay all the bills so I can write movies. 1 don't want any hundred thousand dollar-a-year job as a financial planner or stockbroker. That's my husband's job."

"Leave me alone, you. Only failures marry poor men who beat them and then stay for the free rent."

"Stop sucking away the last recalcitrant ray of my femininity! I'll always have more choices than you." I melted into tears as she twisted her pillow. "I'm outraged you took from me my motherhood, my home, my marriage-any semblance of family support. I didn't know when I married you that the family would become everything and me, the individual, would lose all rights."

"This marriage made me invisible. When I turned to a career there was nothing left standing. There is no career. No one wants to hire me! I've chosen motherhood over a career. I'm tired of reading that only failures marry. Without a loving husband, how can I feel at ease? How can I show my children by example, that I'm worthy of love?"

Ahmed drew me to my feet and slapped me hard across the mouth. "How can you have a career when every time you go out of the house to the work world you're fired for incompetence caused by anger at your boss?"

It was two years since Ahmed's and my divorce, but it was the first time they really talked, knowing they might never meet again to account for what they said.

"I don't want the bloody battlefield of work. I want a husband and my family-but not a bully husband like you were."

"What the hell do you want?"

"To be cherished." I shrugged.

"You've got to give something in a marriage."

"I want to make enough money to buy my own house with my own room and support myself when I'm old and all alone."

I crumpled on the bed. "Commands, commands. There's nothing left inside to barter anymore. I'll always be a lady."

"No. You're a woman." My grandma also screeched at her second husband that she was a lady, and he spat at her like a Marine drill Sergeant that no, she was a woman. A lady is supported by a good provider, her husband or father. A woman supports herself and is alone without a husband or father's money and property to fall back on. Like the book, *Catcher in the Rye*, there was no family to lean back on when the husband left with all the joint bank account money and didn't share community property, didn't even allow the wife to have the children because that was not the custom in his country, even though he made a living in my country. So that was what it was all about—the fall from innocence and not having someone to catch you in the outdoors when you slip, but have not yet fallen. I needed a catcher, and there was no catcher but myself.

The children had curled up on the bed and had fallen asleep. Suddenly I and Ahmed stopped and peered down at the tots sleeping with their thumbs in their mouths.

"You're right. A lady inherits class. She has a husband who makes enough money to support her so she doesn't have to work to live well. A woman earns class."

"So long, kid." Ahmed carried the kids from the bed and shook them awake.

"Just like that? And what do I do with all my fear?"

Ahmed motioned with his thumb up his butt. He looked around for the last time at the cement rectangle where his ex-wife now lived. Sitting behind her table, he ran a comb through his curly chestnut hair and smiled the kind of dimpled smile that any woman would have envied.

"Have you seen my face anywhere?" Ahmed asked.

"Certainly not on airport posters," I joked.

"So your phobia lessened enough for you to take rides to the airport?"

"I was referring to the television news."

Ahmed unzipped his jacket and flung it on the chair. He lighted another cigarette. "How will you remember me?"

"As the man who called me a dirty Jew, a whore even though I was a virgin on my wedding night at the age of twenty-one and totally faithful to you, and took away my babies, my house with the fireplace, all the money in the bank, the Eldorado Cadillac, but not my soul."

My face went numb as I breathed more rapidly with anxiety. Ahmed bent over me, blowing his rancid breath in my face. "Not as the father of your children?"

"It's something I tend to blot out, but it is reality. I never realized in your culture the family was more important than the wife's sanity or health."

Ahmed hiked up his shirt sleeve and smothered his lighted cigarette in his bare armpit.

"I made my presence known in America as I will everywhere on Earth."

Ahmed walked back and forth between my bed covered by my home-sewn quilt tops and the chipped wooden chair. Behind him was a portrait of the children and me in a separate photo, alone. He sat next to me, gave my shoulder a hard squeeze, then leaped, turned, sod thrust his behind in my face.

"Can you find a tail up there?"

I shoved his behind out of my face as I cringed.

"No? No devil's horns? I'm the father of your two children. I'm not an animal."

Ahmed rubbed himself between his thighs. He opened his luggage, shook out a piece of cloth and wrapped his head in a checkered kaffiyeh. Then he hiked up his undershirt. I glared at the shrapnel wounds covering most of his chest and abdomen.

"Even if I screw only one Jew today, it will be worth it." Ahmed fell, draped above the chair as he laughed out loud.

"Goodbye, ax-husband," I spoke without emotion. "And keep an open mind."

"Just who the hell do you think you are?" Ahmed rose, glaring at me with his angry eyes.

"To your own family, you're a hero," I sighed. "Tell your mother I wish her well. My blessings. That's what you get back from the Jew. I'll deal with my anger in private-a woman's way."

I kneeled and kissed the children goodbye once more, straightening their clothing.

"Don't forget to be a doctor." I wiped my tears away and pressed my lips against the children's cheeks. They giggled and hugged me back.

"See my Dancerina doll," Sara chuckled.

"It's beautiful, honey, like the two of you."

This last moment was not the time to spoil it all by breaking down into a crying spell or a tantrum. No, not in front of the children when their last memory in the English language was this moment frozen in time.

"G'bye mommy." Sara's and Davy's voice echoed into the early dawn rain.

"Say, are you kids really my mom and dad reincarnated or maybe my grandparents?" I called to them as Ahmed's car sped away.

I left the light on as I closed the door softly and shuffled barefoot to my rumpled studio couch bed. I turned on a portable battery-run radio and wiped tears on the back of my sleeve. Just as I drew the blankets over my shoulders, the phone rang.

"Yes?"

"This is Hoda."

"What do you want?"

Hoda sighed angrily. "I think you're the most selfish bitch that ever walked to give up custody of your lovely children. Just because you're too lazy and selfish to take care of them. That poor man. I'd never give up my children.

I gasped as if my air was cut off. I fought back the violent shakes, the convulsions. Through trembling head, arms, lips, I tried to speak, unable to raise my voice to Hoda, shrinking with fear of her. But slowly, I spoke with outward calmness, through a cracked voice.

"Hoda, you were married to an engineer who left you a three-thousand square foot house in the suburbs and God knows how much money from his business. Plus you have a job. He didn't put a gun in your head."

"Don't ramble. I can't stand a woman who rambles," Hoda interrupted.

I ignored her. "He let you keep your two daughters. But you wouldn't leave my husband alone. Why didn't you help me woman-to-woman when I begged you not to break up the family? You could have saved my life."

Hoda sighed with impatience. "What kind of a mother are you? Don't you have any soul?"

I hyperventilated and Hoda's breathing was slow, deep and calm. It was clear who was in power.

"And you call me, selfish?" I repeated until Hoda banged down the receiver in my ear.

I hurled the telephone to the floor. At last she was able to release a flood of tears. "Please, please leave me alone. I want a new life, a new family. Leave me alone." If I allowed myself to feel anger or pain, I wouldn't survive it, so I felt only deep fear.

The radio was still playing the 24-hour classical music station. I turned the volume up to comfort herself. Renaissance brass blared forth. then lute strings A slow rendition of "Greensleeves" began to stir as I let go of all feelings and sobbed quietly so the neighbors wouldn't hear.

Silently I watched the dawn brighten the window, then went out without breakfast to look for a job, always putting logic before feeling in order to survive one more day in the search for the road to self-sufficiency, for survival over anxiety, for "making it" financially, and then, only then, could a window of opportunity be allowed to open for love, sweet love and a close-knit family life that never happened, and I speak now in my old age, again pushed back once more to middle age.

I still leave the door open for it now in the sixth decade. It's open and waiting ripe as warm rain. Who can I love, and who will love a penniless old lady with memoirs?

◆   ◆   ◆

18

Friday, Christmas Eve, 1971: Hanukkah, In A Synagogue, After Sabbath Services

The Hollywood garage was mildewed and wreaked of boiled broccoli and beans. Christmas Eve, and I just had to sneak out into the night air and hop a bus uptown. The conservative synagogue was where I went this time to lick my wounds when all else failed.

"Mommy, help me, I've come home again," I sobbed within the synagogue walls. My parents and only sibling had passed away years ago, and I was totally alone, friendless, and in a strange city working at a dead-end minimum-wage job selling display and classified ads on the phone for a small, weekly newspaper. I don't drive and used the bus to get around. A lot my graduate degree in creative writing did for me. Then I began to lose my eyesight in one eye.

Churches were for celebrating when all was fair-weather. But the synagogue was my home and family even though I didn't know anyone when I was troubled. Inside, the 'real' families pared down their loneliness to prayers and cheesecake, I thought. The electricity in the air of a synagogue was the only ghost of a family I had left to cling to as home.

It was the first time I had stepped into a fancy synagogue since September, 1964 when I had stood outside the Syrian synagogue in Brooklyn on the Day of Atonement, three months pregnant. I looked around and saw the same Syrian girls that I had gone to eighth grade class with.

At that time some of the girls from the Syrian clique, the Meegahs, were twenty-three now with children of their own. Syrian girls married young, I surmised. This wasn't 1963. It was 1971, and I was alone, not in Brooklyn near the Sephardic synagogue and memories of Arabic music and the belly dancing I loved to practice at fourteen. I was in a conservative, Ashkenazi synagogue in California, and I was thirty with bags under my eyes that as Betty Davis or Joan Crawford once said in a movie, "only drunken sailors wouldn't notice."

The agoraphobia slowly burned itself out the more I walked and exercised. There still remained the white-outs on the bus, trembling, and anxiety attacks so bad that I wanted to stretch my muscles until they tore to keep from showing passengers how I convulsed with panic disorder.

My hyperinsulinsim required me to stop eating high carbohydrate foods in the morning to stop the trembling from too much insulin and adrenalin being released each time I ate a high carbohydrate meal without first eating protein and Omega 3 oils to slow the absorption of sugar into my bloodstream. I didn't know why food hit me like a bomb until years later. Even high glycemic oatmeal and raisins turned to sugar quickly. When I ate salmon for breakfast and low carbohydrate vegetables such as cauliflower or spinach, the trembling and white outs stopped in due time.

Sabbath services began at eight o'clock that Friday evening. Afterward, an oneg shabbat table was set up laden with egg bread, cakes, pies, cookies and tea.

People filed behind me into the social hall after the prayers for the desert buffet. As I heaped a dab of chocolate mint cheesecake with hot fudge on a paper plate, (bad for my hypoglycemia) Surah, a petite honey blonde slightly older than me, walked up and coaxed me into conversation with a wide smile.

"Going to shul on Christmas Eve? Or is it Hanukah today?"

I swung around. "I get mixed up which is which so I celebrate both. It's synagogue on Hanukah and church on Christmas-just for the pageantry, mind you," she laughed.

"Are you alone?"

"Yes. I'm just going through a divorce." I looked around for a chair. She sat down, balancing the cake and a cup of tea on her lap.

"Hi! I'm Surah. Mind if I join you?"

"Sit down. I could use some company." I ate hurriedly.

"I'm also divorced. My ex-husband was a surgeon. Got two boys, ten and twelve. Where are your kids?"

"I look that old, eh? I mean, old enough to have kids." I looked at her shoes, embarrassed.

"No, not really. How old are you?"

"Thirty."

"I'm thirty four," Surah laughed.

"Your kids live with you?" I sipped her tea.

"No, they live with their father and his new wife. He left me for a twenty-five year old nurse and they have a baby of their own now."

I stared at Surah. "You're the first Jewish lady I met, besides myself whose husband has custody of the kids. Did you give him custody?"

Surah's lips trembled. "Yes. I felt the boys would be better off with their father. After all, he's an established doctor with a new wife and baby. I'm unemployed right now. My diabetes is out of control because of some stupid fruit and nut diet my yoga instructor recommended. I ought to sue him. My ex bought a big house for his new wife. And me? I can only afford a tiny condo."

"Do you have any family?" I looked Surah over from head to toe She appeared well-dressed in black and white velvet, neat pearls.

Surah showed I photos of her children. "My dad is a builder and developer back East. He's got a trust fund for me, so I'm not worried about the pittance alimony I get."

"My husband has custody of my kids, also." I extended my hand and Surah gave it a hearty handshake.

"How come, were you mentally ill or something?" Surah shot back.

"No, I'm not crazy. I just couldn't handle the put-downs and beatings, but he treats the children well. No, he dumped them on his mother to raise. Isn't it awful, but she raises them sell, I hear. Can I believe it when they allow no phone calls from the kids to me, even at my expense?

They won't let me visit the country because I'm Jewish and Jews aren't welcome to roam around Syria these days, so I'm told by that family. Is it true, and even if it isn't, I'm afraid to fly. I'm city-bound by agoraphobia, avoidance personality disorder, and panic disorder."

Surah broke off a hunk of egg bread. "Want some challah and wine?"

"Everyone says my ex is good to the children, but how do I really know? Is it possible to treat them well, but batter me? He could only overprotect them and keep them from independence. Maybe dependence is okay in childhood. Yet how do they learn to be independent later on? How do I know what they're being taught?"

"Why not find out?" I walked with Surah over to the buffet. "Is this the first time you're here?" Surah asked.

"Yes. I've been into religious science for several years. But I've only just returned to Judaism today. I woke up at two in the morning last night after a torrential dream and promised God that I am returning to Judaism right at that moment."

Surah laughed at her. "And what happened?"

"I felt I needed to come home again to loving, open arms, maybe connect with other Jews who might want my friendship. I don't know why I came back. But I have this need at the moment to have a loving family of friends."

"Sounds like you've been just released from a cult."

"No, just a clash of cultures. I tried to narrow some gaps by building bridges, but ended up penniless and with my kids taken by my ex. All I wanted was a loving family."

"Don't we all, honey?" Surah looked me over. "So I'll deprogram you. I just got back from Australia. Worked there for a year in medical records. God, how they treat women! I was homesick."

"Would you like to continue this chat at my place?" I said as she greeted and shook hands with the rabbi on their way out the door.

"Sure. Are you nearby?"

"About two miles." I giggled bashfully. "This is the first time I've invited a human being to my furnished garage without getting date raped. It's so easy making friends with another woman, so safe, I mean. You are straight, aren't you?"

Surah laughed. "Of course. I'm a Jewish mother, isn't that enough?" I asked her for a ride.

"Don't you drive?"

"No, I'm too brain-damaged from an auto accident to learn to drive. I'm afraid I'll get a dizzy spell on the road or a panic attack."

"How on earth do you get around or go to work?"

"I don't get around. I work at home." I cringed.

Bus service was lousy. I brought Surah into my stucco garage studio and draped myself over the sofa bed.

Surah's voice was hoarse and wet. "Here we just met and already we're sisters. Two Yiddish balabustas talking the night away over a dish of almonds. I had a Hannukah bush at my house."

"Why not?" I laughed. "Hey, what about single men at the synagogue?"

Surah pursed her lips. "You must be kidding. A met a guy here who told me his wife was sick with some fatal ailment. After an affair that lasted a year, I found out his wife is healthy. She volunteers here regularly. Try the Reform movement. They're wallowing in divorced men. They have a great singles group."

"So if conservative and reform men have affairs, maybe orthodox men marry for life? What about the Reconstructionist movement? There must be some movement to join where the main are faithful to their wives."

"Forget it," Surah laughed. "Men are genetically programmed to cheat on their wives and eventually divorce them for younger, prettier women with solid jobs or lots of money."

"I can't believe all men are programmed to cheat, or to beat their wives, or to break up the family. Aren't there any marrying kinds who treat their wives with respect and love?"

"Forget California. They're snappy and grouchy. Try Texas."

"You said you already tried Australia."

"He didn't even meet me at the airport. I came back after a year. What could I expect from a pen pal? I fell in love with my pen pal." In my parent's home we spoke no language other than English. Since my American-born parents had been children of European immigrants, what they feared most were foreign accents and tell-tale signs that anyone had looked or sounded different than Americans of middle America. You're dress, language, accent, hair color and anything else about you had to be Standard American English.

So what's an American supposed to look like? We were shown by example. Not the melting-pot or salad bowl Americans. We had to make sure to tint our hair medium ash blonde and to dress conservatively, almost like 17th century Puritans of Cambridge. That's the only way, mom said, to avoid "Having your ears boxed by people that saw you as different." It also meant going to as many different churches and houses of worship as you could attend and to smile at everyone and volunteer to serve the various groups that made the world a kinder and gentler place.

"Don't women make the oddest mistakes in love and work?"

Surah nodded. "Just look at the glow in their wives' eyes. Like they really stick together. You know one Hasidic woman I heard about had seven kids. She-lost her young husband and was frantic for money. The whole Hassidic community pitched in and supported her and her kids so she wouldn't have to work at a degrading job. That's what I call helping your own."

"But not out here. That's back in Brooklyn in the Hasidic neighborhood, right? I mean, I feel better in the Hassidic synagogue, like a family has morals and is looking after me."

"You mean controlling you," Surah said.

"You talk about work being degrading for a wife as if work was hell."

"It is," Surah insisted. "When religion goes the whole family falls apart, doesn't it?"

"One can be moral without being religious," I said. "A lot of people got hurt in the name of religion."

"Do you think religious men ever beat their wives or molest their children?" I inquired.

"Just read the newspapers."

"Did your father treat you like a paper doll?"

"He's loving, doting ... even put my ex through medical school."

My body rocked with tension. "I married outside my religion because I was an abused child searching for passion in creativity."

"Why are you sharing, revealing this to me?"

"When two strangers meet, Surah, they dump on each other if they're that lonely."

"I can't help you."

"'You already have. No matter how far I searched for a drastically different husband, I married a man exactly like my father. It was as if I brought out the same behavior in him. And I related to him as the victimized helpless child."

She hummed. "I had polio as a kid. Then I developed diabetes. Yet I married a doctor because my dad was a famous builder."

"But he left, you for a young nurse."

"And I had that baby my ex and his new wife were having together. My body went through all the upheavals."

"See?" I said hoarsely. "If I had found out you were happily married with your own kids at home to brag about, I'd never have told you my secret. The last thing I need is a friend who's strictly a man's woman."

Surah waved me away. "Don't dump on me. I don't need your secret. There's no space in my life for anyone but winners in the stock market."

"Don't you think I've won the game?" I chuckled. "Would you like to see my movie buff trivia collection? I'm going to be a famous screenwriter someday soon. Do you think I gave up custody of my kids just to be some unemployed shopping bag lady?"

"But you told me in the car nobody's paying you to do anything," Surah chuckled.

"Surah, your children will grow up and spit in your face. Those were the last words my maternal grandfather ever told me when I was fourteen. He never spoke to me much else except that I shouldn't go to college and major in teaching special education."

"No. Yours will."

"Maybe," I scowled. "Or maybe success for a woman is living the lifestyle she chooses. You know why I'm so proud to be a radical feminist?"

I tapped myself on the head. "Reality is all in the brain, sister. Just by the fact that I've refused all employment except writing screenplays and novels shows I'm changing. I'm not standing still by trading class for mass."

Surah leaned forward. "What you and I need, honey, is a date with someone stable."

Tears rolled down my cheeks. "God, Surah I want to get married again. I can't earn a living and make real money at the same time. There has to be some slow-to-anger man out there who will pay my bills and rent so I can become financially secure."

Surah eyed my newspaper on her desk and thumbed through the classified personal ads columns.

"I have this husband-wanted ad running in today's paper." I read it to Surah. "Scorpio. Five feet four. One hundred twelve pounds. College graduate. Seeks marriage-minded man who's safe. Post Office Box Number—". I whispered my ad to her.

"Safe?" She asked.

"Sure. That means he's had a vasectomy or is sterile. I won't get pregnant again.

◆   ◆   ◆

19

Summer of 1973, New York City

Ahmed had dumped the children on his mother and six brothers in Syria and had come back to finish selling his businesses. In the meantime, he offered me a free auto ride back to New York to my brother's house, since I had lost my typist's job for an advertising agency and almost became penniless. After a grueling week's ride with one of his brothers in the front seat and me in the back crying my eyes out because they wouldn't stop at a motel at night, I arrived in New York.

"I never saw a colder family," said Ahmed's brother as they arrived at Benjamin's law office. Samintov greeted me with the stare of an egg-bound tortoise. I was the spitting image of my blue-eyed, freckled, dark auburn-haired father only with hazel green eyes and dark ash brown hair.

"The children have been in Syria for two years and I'm going back to be with my brothers," Ahmed announced stone-faced, to Benjamin. "I'm returning your sister to you to take care of her."

Benjamin was astounded that his bout with liver trouble and diabetes in the hospital resulted in his sister using my two children because I had no home to run back to when marriage got rough. "I'm amazed Samintov never told you of my last hope for bolting with my kids and coming, back to Brooklyn," I reasoned.

"I called Samintov, and asked her to let me have money to get a bus to New York with my kids. But I told her to go on welfare or something and not to bother me because you were so sick. I didn't want to make you feel worse, so I kept my mouth shut," I confessed.

Benjamin agreed. "Yeah, I was sick."

I wished he would have shown more concern when he got well. Only he never knew the kids were sent overseas or that the divorce became final in 1970.

"When our parents died, why'd you make me sign their four-family house over to you when you knew I was going through a divorce in March, 1970?" I asked Benjamin.

"I paid the taxes on it," Benjamin replied. "Besides, someday I'll retire and buy you a house in Florida."

I thought for a moment that the right thing to do would have been to share the house, fifty-fifty when it was sold. But Benjamin, his wife, and their two teenage children were living in it.

"But you own eleven big apartment houses," I commented.

"My wife thought you would ask for money." Benjamin continued his promises and offered me the small apartment in his all-Hassidic building at the standard rent.

"I have to find a job," I protested.

That evening Ahmed, his brother, myself, and Benjamin went to eat in a Syrian Jewish restaurant in the Casbah of Flatbush, the Syrian Jewish and Mizrahi neighborhoods with their ethnic bakeries and restaurants.

I accepted. By nine o'clock that evening, I sat talking to me brother in his new Lincoln Continental. "I'm going up to Maine to see this pen pal of mine. At least he's marriage minded, so he writes."

"Are you coming back to see me again?" Benjamin asked.

I thought of how cold Samintov and me children were to me, and how Benjamin had asked me to sign over me parent's house to him with no compensation for me. "I don't think so. No. I need a loving family," I sighed.

That night Benjamin dropped dead. Samintov blamed I and kicked me ex out of Benjamin's funeral. Samintov said if I didn't visit family and lay the bomb on Benjamin that me kids were sent to Syria by me ex, he wouldn't have been that stressed, but silent.

I couldn't bear going to the funeral. I wanted to remember him the way he was, just like I was with me parents. I sent Ahmed and his brother to Benjamin's funeral and I went out on a date.

Ahmed called me the next day to say held been kicked out of the Jewish funeral service by Samintov and me family.

My pen pal who came to see me in that women's hotel decided not to marry me. In fact the night I was told my brother was dead, I had a date with a penpal from Maine. We went to Egyptian Gardens to watch the bellydancer, and I never told him anything.

I had experienced so much sadness, I didn't want to disturb this crumb of pleasurable music listening moment. Besides, he was reincarnated into a new baby by now, and that conception needed a celebration of freshness and renewal of life once more in the recycling. Life will not be contained. It has been said many times, especially in the cinema. And renewal happens.

"He's probably already reincarnated into somebody's baby. Benjamin will just come back in another body," I told Ahmed. "For every action there's an equal and opposite reaction. For every death there's an immediate rebirth. Back and forth. Contraction and expansion. The law is so simple you can't see it because it's on the tip of your nose."

So Ahmed drove me back to Hollywood and then drove himself back across the country again. Ahmed and his brother left for Syria with the quarter of a million they had from the sale of the restaurant. I got nothing.

By September of 1973 I found myself back in me Hollywood furnished room. Ahmed was in Syria. Benjamin was gone. And Samintov wasn't sharing. I never called Samintov or went back to New York again.

Within a month, I had found a minimum-wage job selling classified ads weekly newspaper and writing a "volunteer" gourmet column. I was just able to pay the rent and eat my fill of brown rice and barley tea. This "me" generation of the early seventies unfolded, only something went wrong with the career track. Nobody promoted creative women without contacts, so the saying goes. I didn't believe it at the time.

The strict macrobiotic vegetarian diet of the Buddhist monks I chose helped me health. After work I'd force myself to walk two or three miles along the beach.

Through belief in reincarnation, letting go, and offering total forgiveness and love to me father, to Benjamin, to all those who touched me life in the past, I was back in graduate film school studying scriptwriting and liberal arts and pursuing archaeology in me spare time.

Little did I realize that what lied ahead was old age job discrimination of screenwriters in the Hollywood arena. Nobody told me in my thirties that by the time I honed my fine art of scriptwriting at fifty-six, that no one would look at my work solely because I was older, even though I would be at the peak of my creativity after sixty.

My health was returning. One day after week of all-consuming loneliness and me first date-at the age of 32 with a 56 year old married engineer who asked me to fellate him (and I ran out of his studio)-I placed a husband-wanted ad in the newspaper.

Out of the 53 or so men who answered me ad in the daily paper, I chose a thirty-five year old never-married appliance repair man who said he was also a double Scorpio interested in psychic phenomena. We met in a Winchell's donuts store for the first time. Three weeks later I asked him whether I could move into his apartment.

He could afford a two-bedroom apartment and I only had a one-room studio. I would have had a whole bedroom all to myself to do my creativity in, something I never had.

As a child I had slept in twin beds in the same room with my brother until I was fourteen and he was twenty-six and finally got married. I hated sharing my bedroom with my older brother, and he probably hated it too, being that he stepped in dog's piss in the living room barefoot one night and wiped his wet foot on my blanket when he thought I was sleeping.

For the first time I had my own bedroom. I'd do anything legal and moral to have my own room, even get married to a man that agreed on separate rooms from the start. How great it is having personal space outside my pockets. All my life I had to sleep in a tiny bedroom with twin beds with my brother until he was 26 and got married and I was 14. No privacy.

Then he brought his wife home to take over that room, and I was kicked to the curb of the living room sofa where the dog slept. I cried a lot, wishing for my own bedroom. Now, at last, I had earned a room of my own at age thirty-three. My new husband, the Anglo Saxon Protestant introvert, fortunately loved to have his own room, too so he could fart as loudly and often as he had to without the raised eyebrows of his new wife. This was what I'd wished for at age twelve—private room of my own, and I finally had one in early middle age. When two introverts marry, privacy is guaranteed.

He paid the rent and assumed all me bills. Eight months later we were married. His name was Eric Auer, and he was a German American farm boy who's mother marched in the Pennsylvania Nazi bund of the thirties. He told me his mother still hated Jews and ran off at the mouth with anti-Semitic jokes that would make the Anti-Defamation League want to punch him in the gut.

I didn't tell my second husband I was Jewish. Not for the first 12 years of the marriage. Eric would watch reels of World War Two Nazi propaganda footage. The torchlight marching in the night, the stirring music. I'd giggle at it in front of him, then sneak off and fear his need for ethnic identity with his American Germanhood.

Then I'd question humanity and secular humanism. Most of all, I believed in Karma. Justice always evens out eventually between the inevitable birth and rebirth going on forever. Why not believe it? My AB positive blood type represented a long line of ancestry that began at the foot of the Himalayas. Everyone told me to get a life. What they really meant is to find values that stand up to the test of time.

It was only when he went out of town for five weeks to company training school did I act on impulse. An ad in the paper caught me eye. There was a Jewish band playing Klezmer music for Israel Independence day.

I was daring. I sneaked into a synagogue and began to cry as the music played. From that moment on, I decided to tell my husband I was Jewish.

I don't give my marriage two months after he finds out, I thought. But I underestimated Eric. He grew closer to me knowing I was Jewish and yet married this German man. Eric was a child of Christian parents, yet a professed atheist. He played the ouja board and spoke to spirit entities and the "force" in the universe and had a terrific sense of inadequacy and inferiority that later led to me becoming a battered wife once more.

Each week we played the Ouja board and asked for spirit messages. There was "Y" the clown, an imp, and his astro-twin spirit, also his spirit guide who spoke to him through the board. One thing they both agreed upon: past lives.

It was a good marriage for the first year. Then Eric became impotent and retired totally to his separate bedroom. From that time on he rarely spoke to me. The only important people in Eric's life was the people he spoke to at work, I thought.

He never spoke to me except in short commands to perform some household chore. Years later, he was still impotent. Nothing had changed in all these decades. I had never worked outside the home. I've traded money for leisure, I pondered. Eric gave me no personal money of me own, just enough grocery money to provide a sparse gruel and vegetarian diet for two and the price of a bus pass.

I spent my days writing countless unpublished plays and novels on my faithful manual portable. I'd think back to the days when the Tunisian I once dated took me to a United Nations party in New York and I walked into an African diplomat's apartment filled with Viennese prostitutes in strapless gowns hopping out of bed and straightening their flowing honey tresses.

I brushed my gray hair then drank a cup of green Magma tea to boost the spirits. I slapped moisturizer on the left side of my cheek that was permanently pleated in a double wrinkle.

I'm tired of three-mile walks through shopping malls with the blue-haired ladies who cough right into my face," I shouted to Eric. He closed the door to drown out me criticism.

Eight of my unpublished novels and sixteen rejected screenplays were piled high on chairs. I had twenty eight dollars in the bank and spent my forty-fifth birthday watching "Revenge of the Stepford Wives" alone. Eric was home watching the football game as he did every weekend since 1974.

He had given me a crockpot for my birthday and told me to go out and enjoy myself in the zoo or park. Am I ever going to make it? I thought as I looked into me own eyes at forty-five. At sixty, I hadn't changed an iota, except for writing more unpublished books, plays, scripts, poems, articles, and drawing lots of pictures.... still so proud, so very proud to be boss of my own creativity.

It feels wonderful to be in charge of what I do each day, who I answer to, and who tells me what I can and cannot create and express, design, innovate, or enjoy. My goal to be creative director moved along nicely. Isn't it wonderful to be boss of your own creativity and have absolutely no one tell you what you can write or what you can put up at your Web site? The air is so fresh and clean at this room at the top.

◆   ◆   ◆

20

My Low-Rent Hollywood Cottage, July 1985

I could never allow my creativity to become a frame that sank from my own sight along with surrounding objects of my youth. Not unless I could know exactly what would be left standing forth as distinctly as a mountain peak. Creativity had become a separate bodily member. What would stand forth and what would vanish? Creativity, those lightning grooves had marked me.

My tiny, ramshackle cottage with its dead lawn stood in a poor neighborhood where children swarmed in the gutter. The streets were littered with overturned garbage cans and empty beer bottles. The street itself left pain standing forth. What if only agony vanished, and within my room, a virtual world bloomed where I could be free to create and express without censure, where I could be boss of my own creativity?

Between the blend of buildings, I built a virtual community of mentors to teach me how to make Tibetan manadalas three dimensional in meditation. Now the three-dimensional mandalas became autobiographies instead of sacred houses of worship. At last, the memoirs became time capsules for distant futures. Salty seas of sanity could be turned into doll houses. I needed to draw silver wakes of grass widening through tide pools and describe in poetry the herringbones of light moving through the fanfolds of my computer screen.

In my house, a kitchen sink faucet dripped water into a greasy pan. Dinner dishes towered in the sink, left to stew overnight as oriental roaches crawled over them. My Radio Shack Model 12 computer stifled itself in the darkening house until Archie, my yellow-naped Amazon parrot, shrieked at the sunset.

Scattered on the floor of my ten-by-ten bedroom was a mound of unpublished novels and a mountain of stage, radio, and screenplays along with books on dramaturgy. Hundreds of dusty, science fiction paperbacks and Trekkie fanzines leaned sloppily in a particle board bookcase.

I drowned out the noisy parrot by flipping my tape recorder to echoes of a mighty Bach Fugue. The music ravaged my room. I glanced at my 46-year old face in the door mirror and stretched the bags under my eyes. Then I ran my fingers through my short, gray hair and twisted in a Tai-Chi-Chuan stance and then a Yoga pose before the mirror to study a still slender figure in sweater and blue jeans.

A concave chest swayed back and the protruding apple belly (from hyperinsulinism) stood forth like a peak from which surrounding objects shrank. It's kinder to say small breasted with tub. I ended up, like most of us, with pendulous pancakes. How calm my shriveled flatness. I couldn't care less about image in a world where image is everything when you look for a job. A social climber might judge me a "B" woman by my hairdo and dress when my prolific achievements on paper-the plays and books—told her I rated an "A."

Who cares about image when you can make your living trading stocks, running up a pittance into the upper middle class? My dream consisted of that three-dimensional visualization as I meditated on-a Tibetan mandala. I worked it over into a three-dimensional building in my mind.

I rasterized any poster image abstract into a three-dimensional pagoda, and the meditation worked wonders for my celebration of joy within, regardless of the surroundings. Again, and again, the cubed mandala became a verbal autobiography, a memoir, and again, a time capsule. Spatial and visual, it became verbal and fleshed out as dialogue.

It took only one ring for me to answer the phone. Noise always shocks me, and I jumped at the sudden jar to outer reality. Introverted feeling is where I'd rather be. There was a moment of static at the other end and a pause of silence.

"Is anybody there?"

I arched an eyebrow mischievously into my forehead and squealed. "Hello? I said hello! Well, I'm hanging up."

As I lowered the phone, a loud voice broke through the static. I whisked the receiver back to my ear. In a thick, Arabic accent, a man's voice repeated.

"Mom?"

"Who?" Nobody had called me mom in more than fifteen years.

"Mommy? This is Fawzi, your son."

"My Davy Joseph?"

"My name's Fawzi Hamid."

"Where are you?"

"Syria."

"You never answered my letters or acknowledged my gifts for the past sixteen years. Did they keep them from you

"I've kept your picture in my wallet since I was four."

"And your sister?"

"Samira's at a friend's house."

"Samira? I named my daughter Sara."

"Mommy, will you help me? I want to live with you. Can you send me to the University near you?"

"Sure, I'll give you anything but the few pennies in my wallet."

I panicked. "I don't have any money. I've been too phobic,—er, sensitive to work for years and don't drive." Oops, I didn't want to take away my choices.

"Can I stay with you?"

"No. My second husband's a miser. He deflects blame on others and beats me down and up like the stock market. This house is too small. It's only big enough for my husband and I. His temper exploded, and he recently put a gun in my head for dramatic effect, I didn't know until much later it was unloaded. He has a short temper like my dad and first husband, your dad. I don't have any money.

He's great to the outside world, a real charmer on his job, helping people. At home he's a tyrant. When I told him you were coming here, he asked for a divorce. Then he changed his mind at the last second. If you ask him for money, he'll give you what he can to make an impression. At home with me, he treats me like he treats his mother. He doesn't like his mother—complains about her all the time. Don't marry a guy who hates his mom."

"What?"

"I'm in an awful marriage with a verbal abuser and twice a year wife-strangler and penniless. I have Mars in Aries in my seventh house of partnerships square my Venus, the planet of love, in Capricorn in my fourth house of home life. That means domestic violence coming at me from the partner.

I'm telling you, he's going to strangle me someday. He's tried it twice already, but I always managed to slip out of his grip and run out of the house yelling, 'wife beater,' and that sets him pacing up and down until he gets calm again. He's afraid the neighbors will hear me when I start to open my mouth to survive."

"I need a place to stay with my father. He's disabled and can't work. My sister's coming also."

"I'll ask Eric, my husband, if he'll kick out his tenant and put you in his rental. It's too bad you have to take care of your father and he has to live in my second husband's house. I thought that man was out of my life, but I guess to you, your father is some god. Do you know I'm Jewish?"

"Are there any Arabs over in your neighborhood who know you?"

"No."

"Don't talk to any Arabs," Fawzi commanded like a controller.

"I've said too much already. Your phone must be bugged," My voice shook.

"Can you send me five hundred dollars?"

"I'll ask my husband to send it to you." I thought to myself, uh, oh, the shake-down is starting. They must think I'm rich. They don't know I've never worked for pay outside the home for any length of time and am penniless and totally dependent on my husband. Fawzi was wrapping my guilt around his little finger.

"I'll let you know when we arrive."

The phone clicked off. I hung up the receiver and hyperventilated with anxiety. I paced the floor, pounded the rug, and stretched, trying to get rid of the adrenaline rush of fear. I'd rather join a skydiving club than have my adult children move their father's world back into my space. What space?

My only privacy in this second marriage lied inside my purse. The house and furniture with all the décor belonged to my second husband, and he didn't let me re-arrange much. I couldn't even put up my original oil paintings on the living room wall.

He tore my drawings down and put up an eye chart so he could exercise his eyes staring at his arrays of paper eye charts pasted up crazily on the walls. Down came my hand-painted mandalas that gave me so much serenity to paint in acrylics.

I was afraid to fly, afraid to travel beyond the city, afraid of people, and afraid to work outside the home-afraid my body would crack before the ideas were hatched. I rose to fear, and shrank at the intensity of my husband's pool of anger.

He always blamed someone else-usually me, for what stressed him out, what went wrong. If only I could escape into that virtual community of mentors I created first on paper, then in my mind, hoping someday I could grow virtual worlds of peace and joy inside my computer in the future. Let me create a heaven, a utopia in virtuality on a computer screen. If only that existed in 1985.

I rose from my bedroom carpet and walked to my husband's bedroom. For the twelve years of our marriage then Eric was impotent and celibate. He always had his own room. My marriage was never consummated after the ceremony. We had lived together for eight months before marriage, and it went along fine with no beatings or scoldings.

After 1976 the put-downs grew worse ... "You're worthless," he would say over and over. "That's why no one wants to hire you. You have no friends." It felt like every abuse dealt on him by his military step father and drill sergeants when he played military now fired at me to bring me down to his level of self-admitted inadequacy and lesser education than I had. I would live with anything in exchange for free rent and food so I could be left in peace to write. Besides, Eric was my only living relative who spoke my language.

What if he knew in 1978 I had joined Mensa, the high IQ society to meet people who might refer me to a job opening?

I knocked on Eric Auer's door. He was annoyed at the disturbance. Eric opened the door a crack, pushing his bald head topped with thick eyeglasses out a sliver.

The bright light from his desk lamp illuminated his face like a skull. The smoke from his soldering iron drifted from his room. Eric, my half-German husband, spent hours as an introverted sensing type, attaching wires and gadgets to a circuit board, building another computer. His own tape recorder was on, playing for his huge collection of old time radio tapes of the Green Hornet.

"Tune me out, I told you. I'm busy, so don't bug me."

Eric shut his door in my face. He turned up the volume of the Green Hornet to drown out my voice. However, I persisted.

"Come on and give me a hug. I have to talk to you. Besides, I need twelve hugs a day."

"Don't nag me." Eric turned up his tape still louder.

"It's important." I whined.

"Oh, give me a break!"

"Not until you give me a connection. How come you only talk to me in commands?" I scratched on his door.

"Quit arguing, for heaven's sake." He pushed me against the wall and shoved me to the floor. Eric's temper went from one to zero in a second For the second time I had married an abuser. This one abused my only half as much as the first. Now there was no way out.

I had become agoraphobic again after the last bout with his pool of anger. I honestly felt I'd go to pieces with stress if someone hired me to work at a job. Yet I kept on trying, in vain, to find a job, somewhere, anywhere, typing all day until my carpal tunnel syndrome welled up.

I planned a quick, simple dinner, and after I'd begin the preparations for the next day's meal. Eric sunk into, his mattress. Then he rose, walked across the room. I was startled when his bedroom door flew open and he followed my into the kitchen.

"You call this fun?" He argued, pointing to the computer he was soldering.

"You can't stand to see me happy. Every time you get your period, you turn into a bitch." He swung his arm across the table and sent the fruits and nuts flying to the parquet floor.

"You clean up this mess," I quivered.

"Mess!" Eric taunted. "What mess? I'll show you what a mess is." He picked up the food and dumped it on the floor.

Then he opened the freezer compartment and pushed out the contents, throwing bags of vegetables on the floor. He took out the newly peeled apples, bobbing in cinnamon puree, and dumped them on the floor. He lifted the cleaver, the milk, the macrobiotic vegetarian Nori rolls-everything that I had spent the night before rosetting and threw them down.

I watched in torturous belief, looking at Eric, the stranger. I looked straight down his heart, feeling the shudder of the shrinking caves of powerlessness beneath my feet. Eric backhanded me, and I jerked my head away-flow mechanics-in the direction of his slap, just as robot-like as his hands dished it out to my mouth. An oval formed on my cheek where his fingers touched.

Gazing into his face was like looking into the glossy side of a toppling wave and seeing myself ready for change, for action. His face extended itself a smooth, shining crystal. In it I saw myself now and as a child on two time planes. Only the future existed now, I thought, as my head sunk back into the turbulent muscles of my neck. The threat of my shadow overwhelmed him.

"Loser! What makes you act that way?" He mouthed the words accusingly. While he pursed his lips and cringed, Eric slowly unbuckled his belt and slipped it off. He wrapped one end around the knuckles of his right hand several times like a phylactery and began slapping the heavy buckle against his left thigh.

Slowly Eric inched closer, trapping me in the corner of my bedroom. I glanced at the bars he put on the window to keep the burglars out which now became my prison.

"You obsolete old biddy," he bellowed. "You forty-six-year old discardable tissue." I flinched as his words ran together, giving birth to a terrifying cadence.

"Crunch ... like the Green Hornet, Batman, Aquaman, Spiderman, Superman, Captain Marvel, the thuds, punches, crunches, shpoofs, foonsps, rained down upon Superwoman as he brought me down to size-his perceived size.

And in the luminous lump of that marriage, I spun in my orbit towards inevitable change, toward growth at last in a dance and a dazzle.

For a moment we both breathed as one-the only time we had touched in years. When Eric was close enough, he finished his sentence by whipping his buckle across my torso. The buckle smashed against my hips, and I sang out. Eric rushed to close the windows.

"Shut up. The neighbors will hear," he whispered. "Why the hell did you wait twelve years before you told me you were Jewish? I didn't marry you that way!"

I turned away, but his second blow stung my spine, almost paralyzing me. I managed to creep across my bedroom. His arm lurched out. And I saw that the anger in his eyes rose and slid like lights dying down a Christmas tree.

I mapped his face without thinking. It was like an electric grid with infinitesimal fluid pulses rising and falling.

"I warned you to tune me out when I'm fiddling with my computer." His voice strained an octave higher. I recoiled at his stale, tired smell.

"I'm sorry, Eric."

I was stung awake to myself and sighed as he left my room. Now I lay in my self-spun thoughts, in the darkness. I saw for the first time that there was an inner template, sight unseen, to my life. I understood that my inner pattern was not yet strong enough to impose itself.

In pockets of memory I caught my own spiraling thoughts. "Need me," I cried in a whisper. Suddenly I saw my whole world from the spinning walls of a bubble as it hung flowing from the red plastic straw in my chocolate soy milk. I sipped sweetness followed by a bottle of mineral water. In my mandala memoirs diary I wrote the words, "like a vale of tears." Then I pictured how I'd look dressed as a Tibetan Buddhist monk.

Another memoir, a tapestry, another autobiography of word and picture went into my time capsule. I liked the idea of making a three dimensional mandala instead of a collage for my memoirs chest. Instead of a hope chest that 1900 brides had for their future memories and possessions, I spun privacy into a time capsule.

Eric, called "the cheapskate" by the women in his family, and "generous Eric" by his brother, whose tuition he paid, slammed his bedroom door and locked it. I returned to my bedroom, tired of always reacting to his answers instead of taking action on my own. "What did I do in a former life?

How and when did I sin to deserve this man the second time around?" I spoke to myself staring in my mirror. Then I added "What if I didn't do anything, if it was a random man I met doing his random actions based on his past, not mine that I fell into? What if nothing compelled or even impelled me to accept all this?

"If he finds out my kids are coming, he'll kick me out of my bedroom and give it to them. I'll have to sleep on the sofa." My memory flashed back to my fourteenth birthday when my brother brought Samintov as a new bride back to his parent's home. And they moved into my bedroom I had shared with my brother since I was nine or ten.

I had cried at having to give up the bedroom I had decorated and taken over when Benjamin married in 1956. Then I had to sleep on the sofa above the linoleum living room floor where my poodle pissed.

I swirled around, twisting my trembling hands. I assumed the Yoga Lotus Position on the cold floor of my room, crying behind closed doors. "Eric doesn't want them.

He'll dread their coming. And I know he'll insist that I sacrifice for them. I'll be worthless again in his eyes." When he heard they were coming, he asked me for a divorce, but at the last minute, he told me that he changed his mind right before I mailed my kids a letter explaining that I would be going through a divorce, would be homeless again, and not to come yet.

I made angry gestures to myself as I rose and stared in the mirror. "Martyr must be the root of the word, mother."

I stuck out my tongue and extended on brittle legs, teasing myself, releasing the hostility at the root of my personality. "Stupid, crazy, loser, selfish. Husbands can be crazy makers, like babies."

The words were the same ones Eric called me whenever we had a fight. The one he aimed at me most often was "loser." His used words as bombs, dropping "loser" on me at least once a week. I rationalized that the names he had called me probably were exactly what he thought of himself. He told me his stepfather and drill sergeant talked to him that way. I believe in reincarnation. What did I do in a former life to be punished this way in this life?

At seven I already knew I didn't want to have children and didn't want to ever fly in a plane. I scribbled it on paper and placed the message in a nightstand drawer to remind myself when I grew up not to take that kind of risk. Only the stock market would be where I would risk everything for the chance to be independent of abuse.

I sat on the edge of my bed—thinking about how the mention of Eric's blue collar repairman's job would cause educated women to walk away from my just as the men walked away from me at college dances when they asked what my father did for a living. "Janitor," I reminisced. They'd bolt from my personal space.

You'd think after all these years your mom would have made it, I thought. How the hell can I bring my kids to a home like this after sixteen years without any letters or calls? I flipped on the television set next to my bed.

The host of a woman's talk show appeared and flashed a toll-free number, and I dialed it. I talked to the host of the TV show about superwomen and working motherhood.

"My body can't take one more punch."

"Have you tried an acupressure massage?"

"No."

"What caused your burnout Are you hitting the wall? How'd you get your hostile personality? You're a bitter old lady."

I tried to respond to the machine gun questions the psychologist aimed at me as the studio audience looked on somebody else's face and somebody else's books.

I squeezed the sweaty phone to my ear. "I'm burned out getting fired from every job for incompetence. Now when I try to work and I'm criticized, my body gives out in total physical collapse. So I can't work. Was it my husband's anger that made me incompetent or my fear of it-since it repeated my father's and brother's anger against my mother during my childhood?"

One of the psychologists on the panel answered my question. "So many working mothers are returning home, burned out from being superwomen. They've had enough. They are dissatisfied with all work and little reward."

The TV host beckoned a second panel psychologist to respond to my call.

"Do you have children?"

"My ex stole my kids."

"Did you ever see a psychiatrist?"

"You've got to be crazy to see one," I laughed. "Housewives enrolled for a master's in counseling are cheaper."

I told the talk show psychologist, "I can't let my kids see how Eric treats me. You hear it, corporate America? Without money, motherhood is the ugliest job in the world." The next morning, I made a pest of myself phoning local radio talk show hosts and hanging up on them (due to my sociophobia) at the moment they announced, "You're on the air."

◆   ◆   ◆

21

My Home, August 1985

Sunday dragged on as empty as a boiled test tube By noon Eric was almost finished working at his computer as he sat in the living room testing towers of software. I stayed in my bedroom, spurred to the height of creativity by Eric's cycle of tranquility. His temper outbursts would coincide with my menstrual cycle.

A week before ovulation, I was at a peak of endurance and could knock off a stage play in the ten days of euphoria before I'd crash into premenstrual syndrome, complain to Eric, and tease out the infant in him.

The phone rang, and I grabbed it. A month passed without her holding a conversation with a single human being—of her choice.

"Mother? It's Fawzi. Samira and I are staying with uncle Tewfik, here in Hollywood. We flew in last night. Can you come over at two o'clock?"

I hadn't seen Tewfik in fifteen years. He was Ahmed's brother who had married an Arab woman and lived fifteen minutes from her. I learned from Fawzi that his father was living with Tewfik for the past five years. I thought he was in Syria raising his kids.

"You were living with your grandmother all these years?"

Fawzi calmed her down, although he barely spoke English. At nineteen, the sheltered, housebound life he and Samira lived in rural Syria frightened them. They agreed to come over.

"It better be important. I'm real busy." Eric looked askance as I hurried over to his computer table.

"My kids are here—with my ex's brother. They got in last night and want me to go over there at two. Can you give me a ride?"

"I guess you must be excited to see them after sixteen years of not having one of your letters answered."

"My son told me he knows nothing of my life."

"Good, keep it that way," Eric sneered as he turned off his computer.

It was a fifteen minute drive to Tewfik's modest home where Ahmed's brother lived with his wife and six children under twelve. I was caught unaware when I learned that Ahmed, now disabled by loss of memory due to brain damage, lived with Tewfik.

I rang the bell while Eric waited in his old VW An obese Arab woman in Islamic dress and a blue rayon headscarf opened the door. Her clothing style contrasted sharply with my sleeveless blouse and white slacks.

I found Tewfik in a neck brace and unemployed. He explained he was going back to Syria because he was unable to find work and had been living on social security for the past four years.

"The sale of my home should bring me a hundred thousand dollars. That will buy me a nice business in Syria."

Soon I got the message. He was looking for someone to dump Ahmed on, now that he was disabled. Ahmed had slipped and fallen, causing him to lose his memory—and he wasn't good for any kind of work except gardening. But he did, get social security also.

Tewfik wasn't planning to take him back to Syria with him. Samira insisted that her father live with her or Fawzi. And since my daughter was going to marry an Arab doctor and move away, that Fawzi now had to care for his father. Now, since Fawzi had never worked, he would need a place to live with an extra bedroom for his father.

I was stunned. The burden of financially supporting my children and my ex husband who came with the package was now thrown on me by the decision of my second husband, an American-born Protestant agnostic.

Fayruze, Tewfik's wife, came back into the living room. I hadn't seen her since I married Tewfik nearly sixteen years before. In all that time she hadn't learned much English, hadn't learned to drive, hadn't left the home by herself.

She was about five years younger than I. Tewfik was an unemployed carpenter and Fayruze had never finished secondary school. The house was crawling with their six boys.

"Where's your husband?"

"He's too shy."

Fayruze peered out her window at Eric listening to the football game on his car radio. She spun around and went to fetch the kids from the backyard.

Samira came out first, a tall, blue-eyed, honey blonde who reminded I of Ahmed with her grandfather's fair coloring. The hug from Samira wasn't warm. The girl was afraid of pressing her body against mine and stuck her rear end out while hugging with her fingers to avoid touching. Samira was a few inches taller than me and wider-boned, like her father's mother.

"Are you happy now?" Fayruze chuckled.

"Oh, yes, she's gorgeous." I looked up to see her son hurrying out of the bathroom. Fawzi looked like a carbon copy of I. The same Semitic face, the same shade in his eyes, the same tone of hair, the same narrow-boned slimness.

They could have passed for twins if I had the bags removed from under her eyes.

"The spitting image of my father. He's probably reincarnated," I said to Fawzi.

"And I look exactly like you," he laughed back.

Fayruze 'Put down a platter of baklawi and kataifi—walnuts in filo dough topped with a sugary cinnamon syrup—and four cups of Turkish coffee. Her smiling eyes raked my girlish figure. "What does your husband do for a living?"

"Technician, he repairs things."

Samira gave her mother a reluctant kiss on-her cheek and Fawzi hurriedly kissed the top of my head.

Even then I felt like an outsider in her children's lives. I was the stranger, the American, the Jew. And they were one big happy Arab family who spoiled her children rotten with lavish gifts. They were the Arab American princesses and princes. I was just the "token" mother.

"My father is a rich man. We had beach houses.-Farm houses. Servants. My father bought us jewelry. Good clothes. We were chauffered everywhere by my six uncles. I went to the best university, majored in engineering," Samira and Fawzi bragged to I over the food.

Then how come your father is a charity case? I thought. How come nobody in this house works? Everybody is grabbing from the American government welfare system? It isn't right. I grew secretly resentful.

"How are things going with you?" Tewfik's eyes narrowed to s I i ts.

"I'm not working either. Can't take the pressure. But at least Eric is supplying the food and shelter."

Tewfik showed her his neck brace. "You should feel sorry for me. I fell and hurt my back."

"I'll go bring Eric in." I rushed out to the car.

"I really don't belong in there as part of your family." Eric argued.

"Neither do I," I added. "But just say hello. I haven't seen my kids in sixteen years. And you are my husband!" Erik pushed himself up the driveway and reluctantly opened the screen door.

"Kids, this is my husband, Eric."

Fawzi and Samira greeted Eric by kissing him on his cheek. Eric shrank back as if violated. Suddenly Tewfik's six children swarmed around Eric.

"Guys don't kiss men in our culture. I'm American. So just a 'hello' is fine." Eric stuttured.

I laughed and Eric finally shook hands with Tewfik.

"How's it going? Did you two have a good trip?"

Fayruze brought out more food. "Would you two like to stay for lunch?"

"No, thanks," Eric motioned to take the food away. "I'm too scared of germs to eat in anyone else's house.

"Phobic. Probably still thinks you people will poison her." Eric laughed wildly.

I interrupted, blushing. "Actually, I'm a strict macrobiotic vegetarian. Just eat Japanese Buddhist monk's food."

"It's kosher," Eric added.

I felt embarrassed. Eric walked around their house, awkwardly. "We have to be going soon."

A month later Eric had kicked his tenant out of his rental, a four-bedroom home and put my children in 'his' house. Although, all the houses he owned were on both our names, Eric made it clear that when he sold a house, the money always was his since he worked and saved. I agreed. If I didn't earn it, it couldn't be mine. In my mind, there was no such thing as community property. I believed deep inside that he would never let me live if I dared to ask for half of the community property. I had been too conditioned by my dad's insistence that the house be on his name only, not on his and mom's names. "She'd only give the house to her father," dad would say. So I automatically reacted as if what I earn was mine and what my husband earned was his. Only I never earned more than a triple digit income each year.

My children insisted their father live with them. Eric lost the rent his former tenant had paid which had been paying off part of the mortgage. Now Eric had to carry most of the mortgage alone. I attributed the destiny to magical thinking—to my astrology chart squares and opposition positions. After all, didn't astrologers prove that men with prominent Aries in their charts were mostly military commanders?

It had to be destiny. There was no free will, or was there? I assumed there was no free will because my parent's sun signs appeared in my astrology chart in the "fourth house of parents and home." No matter how rational I tried to be, the deep fear of astrology as fate and destiny kept me in an aura of dread, anxiety, and tremors.

Tewfik came over without permission and did carpentry work without permission, installed a water softener and hit Eric with the bill, by surprise.

Eric was growing angrier at the way the children were draining his wallet. He was too passive to resist and too aggressive with me because of the guilt he felt.

Fights were growing worse between Eric and I. For the second time he tightened the purse strings, cut down on grocery money he tossed at me on the kitchen table.

Ahmed spoke to Eric now and then, borrowed money from him whenever he saw him, and Eric gave it freely without showing him a trace of reluctance. Then he came home to I and let her have it.

"Why do you give away your power to Ahmed? Can't you see I'm divorced? Why'd you bring that man back into my life?"

"Because I wanted to be a nice guy."

"Can't you see the children only call us when they want money or to use your computer? Why do you give my ex everything he asks for?"

Eric bought Samira a car and Fawzi a car. He bought Ahmed's car for a few thousand dollars and handed the lemon over to Fawzi. It didn't work. Tewfik had convinced Eric he was buying something great. Anyone could wrap Eric around their little finger—but not I. He held out on her—money, sex, conversation and companionship.

"Miser!" I called him.

"When the hell are you gonna make me rich?" He bellowed. When are you going to get a real job or sell that movie of yours?"

I wanted a patron of the arts to endow her. Instead I got back my own father. What karma, I thought. "Mommy!" I cried out and cringed and begged. "Mommy, help me!" But there was no nurturing mommy about.

"Daddy's darling. Generous daddy's darling," Samira sang to her one day, showing the gold bracelets and earrings.

"Nonsense, why would Arabs bomb their own religious society? That lecture is advertised to the public. It might be a unique learning experience. I am a trained anthropologist. And my kids are environmentally Arab."

"We're going someplace else." Fawzi said nervously.

"Okay. I'm full of curiosity. I'll go myself."

He didn't think I would go out at night myself, take the bus all the way to the university and sit there on a Friday night. However, I did. In the middle of the lecture in walked Samira with her fiance, the Arab doctor, Fawzi, and another Arab male friend. They didn't see I and sat on the opposite side of the room.

I looked around. The auditorium was packed with swarthy students from everywhere, a few blonde California coeds. Women in Islamic dress and scarf sat in the back with their infants sleeping or nursing in strollers.

The lecturer, a red-bearded American professor who took an intense liking to Islam spoke about the history of Spain in the golden age of my previous life's ancient roots in Cordoba, which I took personally. It was a glowing lecture about the golden age of Islam in Spain. (He didn't mention the Jews there.)

"But I did. In the middle of the lecture in walked Samira with her fiance, the Arab doctor, Fawzi, and another Arab male friend. They didn't see I and sat on the opposite side of the room.

I looked around. The auditorium was packed with swarthy students from everywhere, a few blonde California coeds. Women in Islamic dress and scarf sat in the back with their infants sleeping or nursing in strollers.

The lecturer, a red-bearded American professor who took an intense liking to Islam spoke about the history of Spain in the golden age of the land's ancient roots in Cordoba, which she took personally. It was a glowing lecture about the golden age of Islam in Spain. (He didn't mention the Jews there.) The professor spoke lavishly about how it's the duty of every Muslim to protect people of other religions living under Islam—and how this worked in medieval times. I stared at my children. During a short break, I went over to them.

Fawzi went into shock. Not only did he show fright at having been caught in a web of lies, but here was his Arab friends with him.

Would I reveal that I am his mother? Would I tell the whole auditorium of Arabs I was a Jew with a Jewish mom and grandma and my children were here as Jews descended from a Jewish mother who turned secular, and now the whole family was posing as Arabs? But how could my children pose as Arabs when their dad is an Arab and I'm a secular American interested in visual anthropology and ice age migrations?

Would I tell all that nobody would recognize the Jewish half of the family or cared outwardly to admit it? Would it have done good to speak out in front of an audience of Muslims and ruin my children's chances for marriage with the Arab of their choice? No. I became the Tibetan Buddhist monk within that I was in another former life and meditated in three dimensions upon a mandala of my mind.

I thought that all those ideas might have been stirring in Fawzi's mind. Maybe. Samira looked down at the floor with her head bowed so low in embarrassment that she nearly fell over. Fawzi's hands shook as I introduced herself as a stranger.

"Well, how are you there? Do you like this lecture so far?"

His two Arab friends looked me over. "I'm into anthropology. Curious. He's a great speaker, isn't he?"

Samira nodded her head and was silent. Fawzi shook all over like he was having a fit.

"It's very good, thank you," Fawzi stammered, trying to shove a lid on his agitation at the sight of his mother among his world of Arab students. I was perceived as the invader of his familiar universe.

I felt like saying to him, haven't you ever seen a Vulcan before? See the pointy ears? But I held my broad smile watching Fawzi fidget.

His Arab friends received me warmly without tension in their interaction. "The speaker has written some excellent articles on Islam's opposition to terrorism."

My goals in life focused on trying to survive. I wanted eagerly the power of financial independence, but had no confidence that anyone would hire me for pay. Nothing I wanted really existed: a job for life, an extroverted, calm stance, or getting affection. To get any of these I had to give someone a job for life, give affection, and spend some time with extroverts. I had no friends at thirteen. I had no friends at thirty-two.

I had no friends at sixty-five plus. Too shy? Maybe. I feared the young were only interested in what they could get from me. Oh, the old lady doesn't need that cash. She's too old and frail to enjoy it for travel. Let's take it from her. That message came from the looks of teenage boys at me on the street. Now and then, they'd pass me and scream "old lady" in my face or laugh at my white hair. I couldn't change it, being allergic to hair tint. The wigs felt hot in the 100 degree summers. I'm allergic to facing life the same as I'm allergic to anesthesia. Why couldn't the young accept me as I am?

The desire seemed to melt and focus on reading about what life was like in the Ice Age, what DNA was like 40,000 years ago, when did my prehistoric ancestors begin to look like I look now? If I couldn't find loving parents in the present, I'd visualize my single common ancestor who lived 21,000 years ago in the Ice Age. I went to the senior centers, but they offered only bingo and crafts. I wanted intellectual stimulation. So I drifted back to 1985 when I was in my mid-forties and thought of Fawzi.

When I was in my mid-forties, I nodded to Fawzi's friend. Current sensation: thick tension. What if they knew all the time I had spent in the disguise of an

Arab wife and passed myself off as one, joining all the Arab social clubs during the two years Ahmed and I lived in Washington, D.C. and while I was a graduate student in journalism?

Even before I had moved to Washington DC in 1965, I went around in New York telling everyone I was Lebanese and Muslim, even letting my first husband put the Muslim religious affiliation on my baby's birth certificate to please Ahmed so he would toss me a crumb of affection which he never did.

It was futile. You can't buy love by changing your ethnic identity, no matter how large and seemingly affectionate the family you marry into, I thought. I needed to become aware of that. I even studied different languages to enjoy ethnic weddings that I hoped I'd be invited to at some future time, but I never did get to be invited to a colorful ethnic, musical wedding where I could dance and smile and be healed by the music.

I've got to get back to my authentic identity, the essence of an introverted feeling type who leaps from intuition to life the way it could be by some divine mind instead of how it is appears in so-called reality. I remembered the time when I had donned the "correct dress code."

The emotional high of knowing you're a Jew and yet posing for seven years as an Arab Muslim in a marriage to an Arab was the familiar excitement I grew on. Like in the old days when her father chased her through the cellar with a hammer or an ax swinging in his fist. It was all a game.

"If I catch you I'll kill you." My father's words never left me for a moment. The career I picked, writing books and plays, had those emotional highs. Career was, like the search for true love, all a random gamble, I thought.

High risk stocks were my fortune. The excitement, the emotional highs had me as much as my drug-free, smokeless, vegetarian lifestyle of Tai Chi Chuan and Yoga, sprouts, and raw veggie juices with the fiber left in.

No other job offered the emotional highs. No other marriage would be so up and down. I thought visually making mandalas three dimension in my meditations. Life was in frames, in pictures, like the rolling of a movie camera.

I even wrote in pictures, in scenes, in frames. Creating was easy. The hard part was organizing and grouping likes together, but the job had to be done, and I did it in a way that made me proud.

It was too easy just being a Jewish wife. I had experience the holocaust and write about her private hell camera frames.

I grinned as I thought about the thrill of knowing I was Jewish and attending all those Arab parties, making friends with all those people who constantly criticized me for the only reason that my great grandparents just happened to be Jewish.

I would come home from that disguise, having lived n their shoes and promptly send off her check, when I had the money, to the World Zionist groups. I even had membership cards in several Sephardic organizations—educational groups for Spanish and oriental Jews. And finally I joined and felt exuberant joy with the Lubavitchers, and studied hard the Hassidic ways with great happiness. I even fantasized what it would be like in the next re-incarnation as a Hassidic man with a long red beard.

Then I'd go home to my Arab husband and try to make him over into a Syrian Jew. It never worked. So I made friends with his Arab friends ... until he threw me out and chased me a block with a carving knife down a dark side street in La Jolla. And still I could find no man who loved me, no daddy, or mommy so nurturing and true. Oh, how sweet it feels to be infantile in old age dreams, but brilliant upon waking.

A lot of time passed until my children called again. Samira had married her doctor friend on Mother's day and didn't invite me to her Islamic wedding she held in the house of my second husband.

Finally I confronted Fawzi about the way he acted at the lecture. "You could have introduced me as your mother instead of cowering in fright."

He shrugged his shoulders. "You can't trust Arabs. If they found out you were Jewish they'd kill my family back in Syria."

"And that's who you stick with—people who would hurt or kill you for having diversity in your ancestry—when you are free to learn from the whole world at the university here?" He withdrew a little more from me.

"The only terrorism I saw was the look of terror on your face when you saw your mother out of her Jewish environment. Only my family has been secular for at least two generations. How'd you like it if you met the Hasid rabbi in our family—your great, great grandfather? I bet you both would have a lot in common to discuss in philosophy, perhaps enjoying a deep conversation about repairing and healing the world."

"My father says he gave you lots of money. He supported you."

"Your father disappeared with a quarter of a million dollars. Who'd he give it to, the Syrian government to release him from spy prison? That's the story I got from your uncle Tewfik before he went back to Syria."

I didn't tell my son that when he was four Ahmed had disappeared with the kids and left me only two shiny quarters on the washing machine.

"Why are you so ashamed that I'm your mother?"

Samira broke her silence as she sat next to Fawzi in my living room. "Look, I don't want to hear about anything Jewish. I want to travel, to visit my real family in Syria. I don't want to be afraid."

"For heaven's sake!" I exploded. "I'm not asking you to be Jewish. You are Jewish—a child of a Jewish mother is Jewish. There's no such thing as fifty percent Jewish. I realize your father is Arab and to you a father is to be respected. He's like Santa Claus to you, but you don't see he dumped you for his mother to rear and took off for America, visiting you only a few times.

"And all this time I thought he was with you in Syria, with his new wife and his mother helping out. He never did marry, I hear now. What a surprise. I heard his mistress followed him to Syria, but he didn't marry her after she called me selfish and accused me of breaking up the family. He wants his freedom, doesn't he?

"You must love your dad. He has few friends, just his children. He's the guy who visited you once every couple of years and brought the sack of gifts and money. And now he's down and out and brain damaged. Love him for me, because he never loved me enough to keep the family together." Samira turned her head away.

I took hold of her hand. "I'm asking you to accept me, to be proud of me. If my kids can't be proud of their mom, then who can I share my success with when I make it? My jealous husband? He's the only child around here who insists on my undivided attention."

"No I won't go to dinner at your Israeli woman friend's house," Samira insisted. "No I won't go back to that Jewish coffee house you took me to."

"Don't you like Klezmer music?" I asked. "It's the Jewish soul that disappeared from Europe. We're disappearing. If only my father didn't chase me with an ax, I wouldn't have been so scared of men wielding weapons and women betraying confidential family therapy. I guess one should never tell best friends family news that should only be reserved for one's therapist. Maybe that's why I write books on how to write attractive family history newsletters."

"You should have thought about that before you married outside your religion," Fawzi said.

"Yes. But now I've returned to Judaism and am doomed to practice it in total isolation from anyone who wants to be close to me. I found out too late it's a family religion; I always thought religion was an individual thing. I keep saying I'm secular, but I need a deity to talk to as if the deity was a loving parent."

"Every religion is a family religion," Samira sighed.

"Do you know why I'm crying?" I said. "When I was your age, Samira, I was so ashamed of being Jewish that I married your father, the Arab. Now, I'm so ashamed of being ashamed. I want to feel proud of myself, proud of my parents. I want to stop being afraid to like myself for what I am. 11

"You can be what you want. Just don't tell me about it," Samira demanded angrily.

I sobbed. "I don't know who I am around you, around Eric, or around your father and his brothers. My Jewish women friends think I'm crazy. They avoid me, embarrass me with their nosiness, their insistence that I tell my life story to every woman I meet in their presence."

"Who else knows about us?" Fawzi asked.

"The whole world. Now I'm ready to drop my need to tell my story. But no one wants to let me change the subject."

"Eric is Christian but doesn't have any interest in a church. He listens to psychics, plays the Ouja board, and likes to read about new age radio shows. He's half English. His father's ancestors have been in America since 1631; half Swiss, Alsatian, or American German with the female side of his family in America for more than two hundred years."

"What does he say?" Samira asked.

"He's an atheist who needs a spiritual connection. So he plays the Ouja boards and goes to Spiritualist mediums for readings, then comes home and tells me what they said about me, all those predictions I don't want to hear about me. He's programming me to succumb to voodoo beliefs in a sense. What they tell me gets into my mind and I live up to it. I don't want to know the future, only the serenity of today. You don't tell scary psychic readings to someone with anxiety disorder unless they calm the person."

"I won't let you ruin my life with my husband."

"Why didn't you invite me to your wedding? What kind of mother's day present was that for me? And you, Fawzi, you called me on mother's day and said you were coming over at two. I had tickets for the theatre. Then you show up at my door and write a note that you'll see me some other time and leave a small gift by my door? I want your friendship, not the trinket.

"On New Year's Eve you said you'll be here. I bought more tickets. Then you call at night to say you're sick. The next day you're not sick. Why are you punishing me so with your promise and your withdrawal? I didn't abandon you, my kids were ripped away with a gun in my head by their father. I never gave my permission for you to leave California."

"My husband and I will come over for dinner" Samira announced."But tell him you're a Spanish Catholic."

"No. Tell him the truth," I said. "He'll only find it out from strangers when he looks for a job and finds out the doctors who do the hiring in this town are frequently Jewish. I know some of them from my synagogue."

"Then you have clout among the Jews?"

"Fawzi knows I have no clout because I have no friends. I rarely leave my house. I dress in white like Emily Dickenson did, and also write poems."

Samira's husband finally found a job back East. They'd be moving in a month. Five friends of theirs from Syria were helping them get settled in the new city.

"How long was he in America before he met you?"

"Three months," Samira answered.

"I've been through this before," I grinned.

"Don't worry," Samira waved. "He'll do what I ask."

"That's just what I said."

"Do you like him?"

"Yes," I smiled, leaning forward as I winked to her daughter. "He's good looking. In fact, he looks so much like your father did when he was also twenty-six."

Ahmed never told his kids that he was a secondary school dropout who worked as a machinist all his life, except when he opened the restaurant. He told them he was an engineer—before the accident. And they believed him.

"My husband was the smartest doctor in his graduating class. He's a genius," Samira boasted.

"He's going to send me through medical school. The university is my whole life. I want to be a doctor so badly," Samira groaned.

"Can I play video games on your computer?" Fawzi begged. "Teach me. I don't know how."

"Eric will teach you. Look at me. I'm forty-six, never been able to learn to drive. I don't have a dime to my name, yet I own three computers. My husband's, mind you."

"I'm getting an "A" in Calculus," Fawzi announced.

"Considering this shell of a family, I'm proud, awfully proud. I only wish you were just as proud of my achievements. I'd rather be admired than loved," I said. "I've given up on love years ago. And you confirmed my feelings when I found you got married on mother's day, that four months passed, and that you already had a miscarriage before I knew the wedding had taken place. Why'd you lie to me and tell me you were going to Hawaii to get married?"

"I didn't want you to spoil…." Samira stifled her sentence.

"Was it because your father was there and everything was done in Arabic?"

"My husband's cousin was there. He invited us to his place after the wedding."

"You went on a three-week honeymoon without telling me. You called your brother everyday. I know you'll never write to me more than once after you move back East."

"That's not true," Samira grinned. "I have a secret. I'm three months pregnant—again. And I'm telling you."

I realized that her grandfather was right. He always told her mother, "Your children will grow up and spit in your face." Children were only lent to parents for a short while. Some "good" kids call and visit a lot. Other kids stay away. Some only come back for money.

My home could never be home for her kids or her husband, any husband. I was always to be the outsider.

"Eric paid a bit of your college tuition. He's given you the shirt off his back."

Samira also feared learning to drive, even after Eric bought her a car.

"You're stepping into my phobic shoes."

"No, I'm not. I married a doctor."

I laughed and gazed at my daughter. "The dream of every American Jewish princess and her mother." At that moment I wished there was a book or gift card I could hand my daughter that had wonderful poetry or lines about mothers and daughters. I remembered my mother slapping me in the nose and the blood gushing out when I was nine. Then what flashed before my eyes were lacey gift cards with the scent of vanilla. What could I give my daughter to remember me fondly?

When she thought of me, it was to hide me from herself and her friends, to hide the fact that my grandma was Jewish. To hide me from her life and her children. At the same time, she asked me to visit. In time, her mother-in-law moved in and took control. My role was never to have control and I didn't want it. I wanted to give the world freedom of choice to express 'itself' creatively in the arts and sciences. My daughter wanted a mother.

Fawzi drank from his can of soda pop and jumped up as the man of the house walked in. Erik heard my remark. "I hate that term."

"I'd go out and dig ditches," Fawzi said, "before I'd let my sister work her way through college or work for a living behind some restaurant counter and be exposed to men's crude passes."

"Would you like to be my father?" I laughed. "Let's have a role reversal party."

I would have given anything for a father who felt so strongly that his daughter shouldn't have to work while going to college or even after it. That's what the father of a princess-by-family-income should be, I thought. A guy who'd go out and bust his butt so his daughter could shop—that's what I want in a husband, but poverty is all I have in my marriage. It's like a childhood dream—to be daddy's darling, where love becomes money a parent offers to a child.

But in the reality I didn't create, I had to work since I was fourteen to earn money for shoes or bus fare or college tuition. I wondered whether if I had married a man of my own background, in time, would I have been allowed to keep my children at least until they went off to college or gotten married?

What would it have been like not to be alone? In all those years I was alone, I thought of them and cherished my private room—until my husband came bursting in with a temper tantrum shoving the door so hard that the doorknob went clear through the wall. The hole in the wall remained for the thirty years we lived in one house.

In 1985, Eric asked me and then my two children, "When are you all getting jobs?" Eric and I never had children. He had a vasectomy long before he met me because he didn't want to pass on his genes for depression and an explosive temper.

"I'm just a shopping bag lady. Forget the saying, 'without a man you're nothing. Without a core identity you're nothing. Will someone please hand me a core identity?"

"Doesn't your husband support you?" Samira sounded just like the 1963 version of her college classmates.

"I get a bed, a bus pass, and enough tofu and rice to keep me revving."

Erik slapped some tofu burgers on the table. "Come and eat. We don't serve pork here. We're all vegetarians." Eric made sure I understood this was his house and he'd decorate it his way. I had to take my paintings off the walls. He said they were junk and cluttered the house. How was I going to express myself without Eric caring? I wrote one book after another. He never read anything I wrote, and it didn't take up space on the walls over the dining room table of our tiny house.

"Just some apple juice, please." This was the first time Fawzi had ever eaten in my space. For months, Samira and Fawzi turned down all attempts I had made to offer them food. I reminded myself that everytime I read the secret diaries that were published of Yiddish women writers in translation, they wrote diaries similar to my diaries, but we were separated by oceans and a century of time.

"Men do have very frail egos," I said. "Have you applied for the loan for school?"

"Yes." Fawzi answered.

"You probably don't know it, but Eric shells out over five thousand dollars a year in mortgage payments for that big four bedroom house of his that you and your father share all by yourselves. It would allow Eric to put away money for my old age if you got yourself a room mate."

"I'll think about it." Fawzi grunted.

"Now that Samira is married, we sure could use that extra two-hundred a month to make our mortgage payments. Eric's just a high-school graduate, not like you studying to be a big aerospace engineer."

"Don't give up your job for me," Eric taunted. "Not unless you want to stay poor, kiddo."

"Fawzi will never work as long as he's going to college," I assumed.

"Why don't you get a job, mom?"

"I've checked out years ago. Twenty years of trying to get a creative job took its toll on by body," I blurted. "I've told you time and time again, my body can't take one more punch."

Eric brought the vegetarian burgers in. "You should go back to school and get a master's in social work."

"Too much unresolved hurt," I mumbled. "But a famous science fiction writer once critiqued one of my stories and called me 'gifted.'"

Eric shouted from the kitchen table. "I call short stories pathological lies." He shoved his face in my lap. "What the hell do you do all day?"

I pointed to the mounds of unpublished novels and plays that filled a couple of rooms. Samira shook her head. "Did you write all this?

◆   ◆   ◆

22

Kitchen Table: Between 1987 and the Present

Finally, I had coaxed Samira and Fawzi to sit at my table and wolf down barley tea and brown rice raisin bread. My macrobiotic vegetarian diet repelled them. The last thing to change when entering a new culture is one's food habits.

Syrian food was what they definitely preferred: rice tossed in melted butter, olive oil, or lamb fat pan drippings with roasted pine nuts, ground spiced lamb and beef fried in fat with yogurt, cracked wheat with mint, parsley and tomato, and a salty salad of goat cheese, greens, cucumbers, and sesame sauce. But they weren't going to get all that fat and salt at my table. Eric ate his heap of brown rice, collard greens, and bowl of stewed lentils and garbanzos covered with roasted sesame seeds and soft, black strands of boiled arame seaweed.

"Really, why on earth did you marry Fawzi's father?" Eric broke his usual silence at the table.

I looked at the faces of my children sitting next to my at the small table. "I'd go to any extreme to be valued, to get attention. My mistake was that I thought in a close-knit family I'd feel important as the matriarch. Instead, I shriveled to dust and the family itself became everything. I didn't realize what happens in a patriarchy—that the rights of the children and male relatives take precedence over the right to be the center attention as the nurtured and cherished wife. I had to grow up fast and see why the children had to come first. It was at the expense of being a bride and a centerpiece.

"Now you are child-free," Eric sneered. "And you have me."

"You've never made me feel good about myself. Every man I rescued became my persecutor. At last I can laugh at my own pain. That's why I write comedy when I feel bad about myself. Because laughing at what I write makes me feet good about myself."

Eric turned on the radio. "So that's why you've refused to work for the past five years?"

"My body checked out, Eric. I've simplified my life."

Samira looked at her watch with impatience. I saw a tinge of shame, the same kind of shame I felt when my mother got arrested for shoplifting and when my dad got arrested for axing my brother's wife over the head. I rationalized that a lot of children aren't happy with the parents they got. My mother said she felt that same shame when her mother gave her away at the age of two to her father when they divorced in 1906.

"Why'd you marry my father?" Samira asked me in a cool voice.

"Do you know what it's like being not only a Jewish American princess—but an uptown New York Jewish American Princess?" My mind drifted to what it would have been like if my ancestors were court Jews in 18th century Germany or Austria and had children who married other court Jews. What if they owned banking houses? Where would they be today, rich in New York or ashes in Auschwitz? What if I had a famous name?

If you had a pedigree, a *yiccus*, you had something to link you back to the great scholars of the Middle Ages if not the ancient Biblical days. All I had was the yearning for that core identity. I wanted relatives that I could show my devout Muslim Syrian children off to, and I didn't have anyone, not even a friend. When I left one city after living there 32 years, there was no one to say goodbye to. Not even the next door neighbor who never once spoke to me. I couldn't force myself to go over there and say, "Hello. It's me." What next? And still, I wished I could reach out and touch a core identity.

Eric stood up and leaned on the back of Samira's chair, rocking it to and fro. "This is a Syrian Princess, right here." He pointed to the top of Samira's head of light brown curls.

"Jewish princesses may get daddy's money, but Syrian princesses stay pregnant and wear scarves on their heads when they marry," Eric laughed. "Haven't you and that doctor husband of yours ever heard of zero population growth?" Eric shuddered. "I think it's disgusting. Why would any woman in my right mind want to have more than one or two children?"

"Hey," I said. "I just remembered why I married their father. I wanted a man like Davy Joseph, a Syrian Jew with a good job in his father's business and a spectacular home with a maid and trips to Florida and ..."

"Why even a Syrian Jew? What not any Jew?" Fawzi asked.

"Because somewhere in an ancient life I was linked to Syria. How else can I explain the feeling of being compelled to break into their clique and the fact that

I was always rejected? Only Syrians brought me bad luck, as if I were cursed by them in some former life and had to give some Syrian man back his two children."

"But we are your children in this reality," Samira said.

"You don't fear your children's father because he has a big family in another country."

"Your father, my first husband put his .38 handgun in my temple and demanded custody of the kids or I'd be killed in 24 hours. It wasn't the first time he tried to murder me. I told the lawyer to give him what he wanted to make him happy. How else could I get that man out of my life? He never abused you. He treated you like royalty. You had a private school, a chauffeur to drive you around, his mother and his brothers at home to raise you. He sent money to you, but I don't understand why he lived in America all these years, and you lived in Syria with his mother, his brothers, and their cousins."

I nodded to Samira. "He led me to believe for 15 years that he lived with you. All the time I didn't know he was living only a 15-minute drive from me with one of his brothers. I thought your father's entire family lived in Syria. How could he have abandoned you to his mother and led me to think he cherished you in person—not just sent money to you and his family in Syria?

"Maybe that's what he did with all the community property, all the money in the joint bank account. He sent it to you. Of course that would be what I would have wanted, but I thought he lived with you in person. I'm shocked. Now, he's come back in poverty, and my second husband has let him move into a house my present husband owns. How strange it all seems so long after a divorce. I understand that unmarried Arab children cannot live alone in an empty house.

Yes, he lives there, but I'm so scared now that his brother also moved in without asking my husband. I feel swept over again. My present husband would never allow you to move into our secular home because it's tiny, less than 950 square feet for two people. The other house is a large four-bedroom.

I understand my husband is letting him live there free and is paying two mortgages because he feels sorry for your father now that he has come back from his last visit to Syria so physically and mentally disabled. I understand that for some reason he was beaten there for living in America. And I can't understand why you still choose to live with that side of family belonging to a wife beater. Then on the other hand, my second husband is American, but still is a verbal abuser. No matter how far I've traveled in years and diverse ethnic men I've met, I still end up marrying a man exactly like my father in so many ways such as personality preferences."

Eric later entered the room where my children and I were having a conversation. He carried his radio and finally clicked off his favorite mind-body-spirit program. "Tell them about the ghost that came on the Ouija board or in your dream, whatever it was. Show your kids who told you about your future if you decided to have kids in the first place," Eric stuttered.

"When I was seven years old, a spirit guide came to me in a dream and told me never to have children and never to ride in an airplane." I took a sip of barley tea. "See what happened when I had the children? If you think I'll ever go near and airplane, you're crazy."

"Yet I wonder if it wasn't just my imagination? My mother always warned me about the hard labor she had with her own babies. The doctor told her he was going to cut the baby in three pieces to pull it out. And she screamed as the ether cone descended on her face. It seared me so much I really never wanted to get close to any man. I was seared of sex. And I just wanted a career.

"Then I went to a rebirthing session and went through it all over again to get over the trauma. Babies do remember. Mom told me all the details since I was three and then again at five and at seven and nine and eleven and on and on. Why? I had two children with a four-hour labor. It was nothing to be scared for. Knock on wood. And pretend to spit three times as the Hasidim do."

Fawzi left the table. "I can't stand that kind of talk. It's getting too deep, too serious for me." As usual, he tried to stifle me by turning up the radio louder.

"When did you first know my father was going to leave you?" Samira ate a handful of raisins.

"I was sweeping the restaurant floor when I told him I had organized the area's first women's lib consciousness-raising group, and they wanted to have a meeting in the restaurant. He shouted to a customer that all feminists should be marched out and shot. The young, male customer looked over at me. But I cast my eyes downward and went on with my sweeping without saying a word."

Eric grew restless. "That's a bunch of bull. Women's lib. Made up of——." With supernal mind, he controlled himself from uttering any epithets in public.

"How have you been, Eric?" Samira broke in.

He frowned as if nauseous. "This house is such a mess." Eric swept some crumbs from the kitchen table onto his palm. "You'll have to excuse the way the floor looks. My wife is such a lousy housekeeper."

"Take it easy, we don't notice it," Fawzi laughed nervously.

I hurried into the living room to escape criticism. "Nobody's noticed this." I pointed to a framed certificate on my living room wall. "It says I'm listed in 'Who's Who of International Authors.' Isn't that great?"

"But did you make any cold cash lately?" Eric snapped.

"Two years ago I published five books."

Eric rubbed his fingers together to signify money. "Aw, my books are already out of print. None of them sold enough copies to put cash in my wallet. Without me, I know I'd be a homeless hag and I am in my old age."

"I told you kids what I am," I replied. "It's okay to fail or to simplify your life. You grow a little more with each change."

Eric sat down in front of his computer in the living room. "Money talks."

"Eric expects me to become the engineer he wanted to be. But his high school counselor told him not to aim that high—that his I.Q., was too low. He only found out in his late forties that IQ tests don't tell the whole picture."

"Intelligence is still mostly genetic," Eric protested. "If you're so rich in ideas, why aren't you smart, I?"

"All my life," I whined, "the types of religious leaders I sought out drummed into my head that prosperity was my divine right. I kept saying business was great, life was wonderful, and people were good."

I sat on the sofa between Fawzi and Samira. "But as I stepped up to the wall, I kept hitting my face into a ton of bricks. Then I'd get back up, smile and insist I'm rich. I was taught to fake it until you make it. Live as the rich do until you become like them through networking with rich contacts."

"But you can't even drive a car," Eric interrupted.

I strained to smile. "I took a bus to the richest neighborhood and walked along those streets as if I really belonged there. I've lived my passion. There's one belief I will never let die: if you live your passion, success will come to you because you're throwing your whole self into the production."

"That's nonsense," Eric said.

I wrote about successful women who change for the better, but I sent my books to critics who always shot them down.

My eyes sparkled. "Everything I set free in this house always returns."

"If it doesn't," Eric laughed, "I hunt it down and kill it. Naw, I'm just joking."

"Your jokes are always sadistic, and make me cry with a feeling that I'm still being denied pleasure, travel, and food," I sighed. "You have in your fifth house of Romance and creativity, Saturn in Aries opposite your eleventh house of groups and friends with Mars there in Libra. Yet being married to a misogynist makes a lot of material to write about. My whole life is one book after another and one dozen plays, at least."

Samira rubbed her eyes. "I weigh nearly a hundred and seventy one pounds. Just a few months ago I was a slim, new bride. Did I build this wall around me just to get out of working? Am I that much my own mother? No matter how far I run—even marrying a doctor while you married a blue-collar worker—am I really you? Mom, are we in competition?"

"I wished you were a superwoman instead of a housewife of a rich doctor. No, I don't wish you became a doctor just because I never finished my doctorate in archaeology. As long as you're a doctor's wife and he supports you, you won't be asking my husband to pay for your education. It would deprive me of any money held set aside for my old age. I wish I were a superwoman," I said ... "and not dependent on one man for my life."

"You are." Samira laughed.

"I'm too determined to be boss of my own creativity to please the authority figures out there," I sobbed. "No matter how hard I try to make my work perfect, they still say I've done something bad and won't pay me for my sweat. So, if I refuse to believe in scarcity and please only myself, I'll make it."

"You don't have to please the whole damn world," Eric said.

"How muck, easier I have it," Samira boasted. "I have to worry about pleasing only one man."

I thought a moment. "Maybe that's why I checked out. Only I chose Eric, probably because he's as familiar to me as my father."

Eric stood up. "Only failures marry. That's what a women's libber told me back in the seventies, Fawzi. Did you know that secret about women? Each time a woman's job gets too familiar, too boring, or in danger, she has a baby to tell her she can create something original without a glass ceiling.

"Those who succeed in their careers don't feel they have to bolt to grassy oases for nourishment and reward. Some feel that husbands and children come and go, but jobs are forever. And others feel that jobs are disposed of easily, but children and progeny are lasting and will colonize other galaxies and end up being for-ever—until the universe contracts and then will be reborn again. It all begins again with different scenarios."

"Twenty-two years has passed since Samira was born," I said. "I've earned the right to choose to be a full-time housewife and get paid for it."

Eric trembled. "Not with me, you don't. Remember how cheap—how much a miser I am. Ask my family they will all agree. Look at me, my car, and my house. Now that's cheap."

"You see, kids? Eric's my inspiration to create best-sellers and screenplays. Unless he whips me into motivation to achieve, I'd be just like you, Samira, a doctor's wife languishing in pregnancy naps."

"Did you Arabs ever hear of women's lib?" Eric smiled.

"Women's what?" Samira asked.

"He thinks his lashing scorpion will flog me into learned helplessness, that I'll be so browbeaten by his misogyny I'll be unable to create wombs in men."

Eric was calm. "Keep trying, kiddo. You can only get better. I know how much you want to get rich."

"I've got a great new agent. And I'm taking a film script writing class With a real, live producer."

"You're too old. Nobody will buy your stuff. They won't touch you because you're too old."

I clenched my fists. "I'm hooked on the adrenaline rush, the passion of creating reality from my own visions and the dreams of people whose lives I touch. The movies in my head talk to the world. How can Eric ask me to spend my gray-haired years filing for five bucks an hour?"

"There's gold in computers."

"File, sort, process, or calculate, it is all that computers do Eric, just file away records."

"But they're okay when I let you revise your manuscripts on them, eh?"

Eric extended his arms to show how big a problem he had. "You're a dreamer wasting your last years." I closed my eyes at him.

He turned to Fawzi to form an old boy's network. "I mean, your mother's got a good mind. I's been in Mensa for the past ten years. I could have done something practical. Financial planners can make fifty thousand a year."

"I have this terrific story in my head," I hyperventilated. "New York. Nineteen ten. An immigrant guy starts a Jewish newspaper in Spanish written with the Hebrew alphabet. It' a true story."

"Go ahead and write it, mom," Samira cut in.

"His name was Moise Salomon Gadol. He fought unemployment with his newspaper," I added. "Nobody else was looking at poverty-stricken Sephardic Jews who came from Greece and spoke a Spanish dialect. Most of the labor movements were directed towards helping the Yiddish speakers on New York's lower East side."

"Yes, write it," Eric bellowed, turning to Samira. "I can't get any other housework out of my wife."

"I deserve to have a maid for housework come in twice a week. If I were a J.A.P. married to a rich lawyer, I'd have my three kids and a live-in maid and a big house with a pool and …"

Eric pounded his fist against the wall. "But you're not. You're married to German thrift."

"Not Irish wit or Jewish humor!" I continued. "Writing is my only connection to the Jewish people."

"I'm against all religions," Eric scowled. "They only make wars. I, you know that once your children move away they'll never speak to you again because you're Jewish."

"I'm scared of Jews," Samira whispered. "If my Arab friends and relatives find out my mother was Jewish, do you know what will happen to the whole family over there?"

"Let's face it," I said. "You two only visit me when you need something fixed, some money, or to use my computer." Eric turned on his computer.

"Religion is an addictive habit," Eric continued. "You see your writing as religion. I believe in poltergeists and Ouija board spirits, in reincarnation. And Karma's gonna get ya if you don't watch out."

"I need a spiritual connection to something, Eric," I pleaded. "I'm so lonely and so choosy about how I prioritize my time. What I need most is two religions. One isn't enough. I need all the holidays. I need to feel included in two strong religions, maybe more. The mystic and meditation, the Yoga and Tai Chi Chuan have to be part of it all for the sake of my need to unwind and celebrate joy, charity, kindness, and being at one with everything in the universe. We all go to the same place."

Eric stuck his nose in the air. "Frankly, any religion that would separate the sexes, cut a man's genitals, or 'nail' a man on a phallic symbol and then wipe out your guilt at murdering him by inventing the story that his carcass is taking away the sins of the world is barbarian stone age shucks. I bet the fourth-century Romans invented a religion to make sure people paid enough taxes to feed their soldiers and keep the incoming peoples subdued. It's about control by guilt, fear, or anger with the promise of love. Can you imagine drinking someone's blood symbolically to wash away your missing the mark? Think how stone-age it sounds, how cannibal. It's like eating the brains of a smart aleck to get his sharp mind."

"Most religions still put women down because they were recorded in times when women were property of men, like cows," I added.

"Religion belongs in the stone age," Eric said. "Too bad the human brain is automatically wired to need religion. Without it, how can the mind heal the body?"

"Along with intolerance," I agreed. "Then how else can I feel good about myself by getting in touch with my roots?"

"Stop hating yourself and start being proud of me. Look at all I've done for you. Another man would have kicked you out long age," Eric ruled. "Hey, kid. You're going to make it big. And I'm going to win the California lottery."

Is that the odds I have against me of making it?" I plopped down cross-legged on the carpet. "Hope is an excuse for doing nothing, Eric."

Tears rolled down my face. "I couldn't be a superwoman and raise kids at the same time. So I gave up the kids and chose to be the superwoman. Then nothing happened in my career. Nothing. And I can never get my kids back the way they were—close to me, like me. I never knew a woman can have it all, but just at different decades of life."

"You wouldn't ever work for me," Eric roared. "How on earth could you work for anybody out there?"

"Holding the lamp over your motorcycle in a cold garage while you complain for hours—or scrubbing the bird droppings off the front walk on a hot day? Unpaid labor? Sorting your filthy underwear in the laundry? You're the only one who wastes my good idea time, Eric."

"You've never done what I asked. No wonder everybody else fired you from work. You're a born loser."

"All I want is to be my own boss. What a marriage. Two people living alone in one, tiny divided house with only the husband giving orders to the wife. Sound familiar, Eric? What's the alternative? Sleeping under the stars as a bag lady and getting raped and cut up in stinky California beach rest rooms as a way of relieving your tooth pain?"

"Mother, mother," Fawzi interrupted. "Are you happy?"

I got up and began to clear the dishes and empty snack containers from the table. Fawzi and Samira followed me into the kitchen. "We've got to say goodnight."

"You bet I'm happy, kids," I shouted over the rushing water in the sink.

"It was all worth it. I'm so much stronger now. These experiences have made me grow so vibrantly alive with creativity that for the first time in my life I have the time to put my hidden passion into words and sculpture."

Samira and Fawzi hugged their mother. "I hope you're not being worn down," Samira said.

"No, I'm being built up."

"What's that?"

"My Star of David," I said. "Too bad I don't have anyone to pass it on to in the next generation."

"I'll take it," Fawzi sighed. I knew he'd never show it to his Arab Muslim wife from Kuwait.

I put the gold star and chain into his palm. "If you really don't want it, please give it back because it's real gold worth a hundred dollars."

"I'll keep it," Fawzi put it around his neck, inside his shirt.

"Thanks. but I bet you'll take it off when you get home, and put it in a drawer because all your friends are from Syria. Right?"

Fawzi smiled.

"We have similar horoscopes and blood types, so we need to eat a vegetarian diet and take enough vitamins and minerals." I grinned at my son.

The kids left. Eric opened the door for them and put the porch light on. "Drive safely, kids." He switched the light off to save on the electricity bill even before their car pulled out of the driveway.

When they were alone, Eric put his arms around I for a moment. He didn't look at my, but at Archie, the parrot.

"They're looking at us," Eric smiled with his head turned at a right angle away from I as he gave me a weak hug. He patted my nervously on the back with the tips of his bony fingers. This was the only body contact I ever got from him.

"Nobody's looking at us." I repeated as I had for a dozen years of their marriage.

"You're going to make it, kid," he said over again, using the same phrases every time they spoke with each other.

"And making it no longer depends on somebody else buying it." I kissed the air, since Eric had never kissed my on the mouth. "Making it means doing it."

"And doing it is free therapy," Eric laughed

"Sure, why not, if it makes me stronger?"

"Free, is the word I'm looking for," Eric added.

"How do you expect to eat?" Eric folded his arms and legs and leaned against the living room wall.

"From the same worn crockpot where you get your own stew," I laughed. "You thirty-thousand dollar-a-year repairman!"

"Where do you think your next pair of shoes is coming from?" Eric grumbled. "Don't look at me, you parasite—just like your daughter. You're not a cripple. I don't want any cripple for a wife. If you want money, go out and earn it like everybody else. If you can't pull your own weight around me, the door's open."

"But Eric," I squeaked. "I've ended up in the hospital eight times when I tried to please that director of public relations. He said the client didn't like the way I wrote those press releases. I spent weeks re-writing. They wouldn't even pay me the lousy fifty dollars per press release. A man would have charged them a lot more."

"Work, like everybody else," Eric said as his face reddened.

"My body collapses when I try to work for anybody. It's the criticism that's the killer. I can't please anybody enough to get paid for my labor. And I really roll that boulder uphill each time. But it always comes rolling down on me."

"Jerk! You can spend ten hours a day on my computer writing screenplays or novels, you stupid stump, and feel fine afterward."

"I've joined Jerks Anonymous. Does that please you, Eric? Maybe you'd like a membership card also?" I'm tired of revising my work for others for a pittance, giving away all the rights, and doing my thing while the buyers of my creativity become rich producing and telling me what to revise over and over for peanuts, for nothing. I want to publish my own stuff and write it the way it ought to be. When I revise my own stuff, the joy will come to me through my audience, not through some animator who needs a slave writer quick and cheap."

Eric hid his anger behind high-pitched laughter. "Did you ever meet a guy as immature as I am?"

"Did you ever meet a woman as adolescent as I am? I can't leave my college campus as long as there are free lectures.

"Once I tried to teach at a two-year college, Eric. But I felt I belonged in the student's seat. One student fell asleep while I was ranting how great it was to write ad copy. There was nothing left to say to the class."

Eric arched his back. "It cost me eighty dollars to pay for your community college instructor's credential. Who paid for your Master's degree in English?"

"I earned the money working as a teacher's aide. The 50 dollars a week you gave me to pay for food for the both of us didn't pay for my graduate degree."

"Then why won't you work?"

"Can you picture a teacher who's afraid to speak in front of people? All my life I was the student. My mind is open to learning what's important to me from others. But a minute later, I've forgotten ninety percent of what I've heard or read. There was nothing inside me left to tell the students."

"Except your false fears," Eric said.

"Do you want me to be proud of you as my husband? Then support your wife like a man. Both of us are products of the forties and fifties. We're imprinted. A lady marries a good provider and he takes care of her bills. A woman isn't as lucky. She works for a living until she's terminated when she gets old or slows down. That why women are like computers."

"I should live so long. That's a Yiddish inclination isn't it? Is that what they call it, an inclination? Here's another one—my eye. Don't New Yorkers say, 'my eye'? What does 'my eye' mean? From what language did it come?"

Eric began to unbuckle his belt, a sign that a beating was coming if I didn't cool it. I took the hint and left. Eric followed me. "What about my needs?"

"You never told me you had any. I mean you never kissed me on the back of my neck." Eric piled boxes in the family room, old papers and brooms. I longed to decorate it to look pretty. Now I stared at that room that hid the green view of the backyard outside.

"Well I have a bomb to lay on you," Eric shoved my against the bathroom sink. "I'm getting a facelift tomorrow. If I don't look young enough, I'll get shoved off my job. Then who'd pay the bills that allow you to look as white-haired and wrinkled as you let yourself be?"

I smiled. "If it makes you feel good about yourself, go for it. As a recluse, I don't need an image to express myself."

"Don't give me that new age Aquarian crap." He turned on the faucet and dipped his fingers in it. Then he flung drops of cold water in my face.

"Turn on your computer, Eric. I want to see that new computer program of yours."

Eric looked at the leaking stains or the bathroom ceiling. "Oh, no, fixing that roof will cost me a fortune."

He lost his trail of thought and turned off the water. I leaned over the tub and belched in relief.

"Turn on the computer in your room." In a minute Eric booted up his desktop IBM clone.

"See how good I am to you? I bought you a two-thousand dollar computer so you could write your books and make me rich."

He slipped a software disc into the machine, impatient for. the whirring computer to accept his commands, to be under his control. He tried to hurry it up. But the screen swirled into a spotty spin of confusion.

"Techno-stress. That's what we're suffering from, Eric. You expect me to respond to your orders like a computer. And when I don't, you lose your patience. Do you know why you're so insensitive to my feelings? Women are as interchangeable to you as computer peripherals."

He slammed the door, drowning but my shrill voice.

"Give me the right to tell you my feelings, Eric. I promise I won't accuse you anymore. Just accept the fact that I have feelings different from yours."

I stopped begging. "I can't ever get through to your passive-aggressive, withdrawing personality," I muttered. "It drives me wild!"

A moment later, now calm as if nothing happened, Eric called to my. "Come see my new modem."

"Why don't I go in my room and put on my computer?" I knew he was into his usual denial now. "Then your computer can talk to my computer the rest of the evening. Sounds like fun, eh?"

"Oh, it's going to run up the electricity bill," Eric complained.

"Come on, only a few minutes. Then we'll play the Ouija board. You like that, don't you?"

Eric hesitated. "Just five minutes. Then I have to work out my software program. I promised someone at work I'd volunteer take a bug out of the damn thing."

"Well, you're not getting paid for it."

I scampered like a child to my room and booted up Eric's other computer. I slipped aside a page from the new screenplay I'd been writing on it. "They don't make 'em like you, anymore, or like me," I said to my old, manual typewriter beside my desk.

The modem flashed red lights. Eric keyboarded on his computer, "I'm moving back to Maryland. I want a bigger house."

His message came up on my computer screen. As soon as he paused for my reply, I typed back, "What will become of me when I'm an old lady that everybody spits at?"

He paused and keyboarded, "We can get a house with a big yard real cheap back East, and I can walk in the woods to experience the change of seasons. I'm a cold-weather guy."

Then I typed back, "What if I slip and fall on the ice and break a hip in those snowy winters when I'm old with hollow bones? I'm a tropical fiesta person who loves the swaying palms and the long walks on the beaches at sunset. I demand Romance."

Eric read my message and entered in capital letters, "TAKE IT OR LEAVE IT. You don't slip and fall to break a hip. The hip gives way first from bone loss if you don't take your natural progesterone, and then you fall. I read all this in my holistic health books and magazines. If I'm good for something, it's guarding the money and nutrition of this household."

I smiled with predictability at Eric's ways. He seemed to grow on my after all those years of marriage. I needed to escape to my world, and so clicked on my television set. The bed was warm and soft. I rested against a mountain of pillows and shifted my remote control device until *Lifestyles of the Rich and Famous* came on the screen. At last I was at peace.

Eric was in my room within five minutes to say goodnight as he had every evening since 1974. He opened the door without knocking and stood with slumped shoulders by my bedside.

"Stand up, if you want your good-night hug. I'm too tired to bend my aching back."

I jumped up not to miss my only chance to get five seconds of body contact. He gave me a brief, finger-tapping hug. Eric's head towered over mine by a foot. He was watching the television set, hypnotized by the flashing patterns.

"Don't you ever look at me when you hug me? Can't you rub my back smoothly instead of that nervous finger patting?"

"I can't be perfect. You're not my ideal, either."

"I'm sorry, Eric. That radio psychologist made me promise not to criticize you for not being a perfect prince."

"I promise next Saturday night I'll give you a hug. I've run out of gas."

"Next Saturday night will be another excuse, just like it always has been. I need my twelve hugs a day." I squirmed in his grip. As soon as he recognized my neediness, Eric danced away. I called him the take-away-man. Whatever he gave, he quickly took away something more valuable.

He peered on my desk and saw a file marked "Science Fiction."

"Ever notice how fat and ugly the women are who read and write science fiction and how slender and glamorous the Romance writers are?"

"Not really."

Eric insisted. "Why don't you write Romance?"

"I have skin hunger," I whined in a New York accent. "And I want the whole world to know the last time I had sex in my early thirties was in 1976 after only less than a year of marriage. Nobody really cares, either."

"Neither do I care."

Eric closed my bedroom door and hurried into his own room, sliding the deadbolt lock on his bedroom door. I climbed back under the covers and watched the rest of the television show.

Love had reeled down the most revolutionary road. At last I had taught myself to set limits. I wrote with the passion of a woman who faced my broken-ness, who had finally broadcasted in a loud voice: I want. I need.

No longer was I concealed from myself or the world. By five the next morning I was back at the computer writing my new "Woman in Space" series that would never see daylight outside my shelf, rejected too many times to count by those who count.

The blank page glared before my as I typed my opening lines: Right Brain-Left Brain Couples. Due to different ways of solving problems, he had a career in hard science. My career was in poetry therapy. Title: Psyche Squad: Poetry Therapist in Space. Then I moved to monologues and then focused on memoirs: Time capsules. Life stories that had impact and held universal appeal.

I loved to work on many imaginative levels at one time. Poetry put me into a trance where I suspended my normal way of thinking. With poetry as therapy, I changed my usual habits. I never thought of having an affair. I'd just write a romance novel when I needed affection. When I tried to give it, rejection was plain. So I wrote it and set the romance in ancient Neapolis, near Rome during the Republic in 150 BCE.

Each time I read or wrote a poem, I protected myself. I could never resolve emotional problems by steely logic. I had to use poetry. Every dream I had, every fear was a product of a conflict and my attempt to resolve it. So I tried a different solution, rose from my own ashes, and soared in moving between ethnic music of all over the world, visual art, and poetry as personal broadcast networks, monologues, plays, and memoirs.

These were ideas for a new play/novel package. I wrote until lunch time when the house was sunny and quiet. I felt good inside and decided to try my luck at imagining what it would be like to study to be a Poetry Therapist for awhile until I understood how one might function in space married to a left-brained man.

I knew my book and screenplay had to wipe away rigidity and finality in the human condition before I could put my healing sounds of world music along with poetry as my personal meditation, my own therapy in space, or it could succeed in visual form.

The evening of my forty-seventh birthday, after baring my soul on paper, I knew I had leaped from the treadmill of submission, rage and guilt. By fifty-six, I began to be able to write what I wanted about the subject I desired and revise under my own direction, answering to no one other than my intended audience.

Threats were meaningless. I had control over poverty, but I earned not one thin dime. Joy existed in writing what held importance. My ability to react, then to act, was renewed as my novel, my plays, and my book of memoirs began to raise and rebuild my own inner laughing wall.

It wasn't necessary to bolt. I had gained insight into myself and no longer thought with the logic of the psychically impaled. I would never again retreat from knowledge to a knotted life.

The act of writing my plays, novels, stories, poetry, memoirs or the sequels to the novels and the how-to books gave me eyes, mind, and will. No more would I trap myself between my family's love and their ridicule.

I had become the character I hated most and loved most. And when I saw what I had done, I contested the origins, re-inventions, and recycling of my own identity. In the mystic, truth became concrete. In the abstract, intuition evolved into resource.

Yet—if I were to create wombs in men, caverns of deep, physical thinking, then I would risk life for one moment of absolute power. You see me in a pink mist, my face blurred by your anger and my fear of your anger. You gaze with those unfocused eyes that forever stare at a point above my shoulders. You taunt me with your wicked mouth and swing your brittle legs like fascists in pantyhose. I only seek to find all the universals in me that make sense to you. The search for identity is only one part of the whole universal shebang.

Men are what they are, I say. Women, by where their husbands itch, are judged at work by wives who marry rich. "And what does your father do?," say young men before they dance. Will he set me up in business? Will he pay to take a chance?

The dusty years rolled by. These memoirs give me strength now that I can work for my next meal, twist through sieves, or tap a time capsule for nourishment.

Growing up is about "always having to revise." And with blessed retirement, came the opportunity as creative director to revise only under my own direction. I, at last, remain, boss of my own creativity.

Collegiate young men today in some circles still ask women under 25, "What does your father do for a living?" Why don't they simply ask, "What do you do—or plan to do?" Single people in their early to mid-thirties do ask one another "What kind of work do you do?"

The younger men may seem more interested in what a woman's father does, if she is to be the future mother of his children and a stay-at-home wife. It's as if the younger man is asking whether the young woman's father will consider setting him up in business, paying for his graduate work, or helping him financially.

And married women, particularly stay-at-home wives, at parties still ask, and what does your husband do? By asking, some women feel diminished, that they weren't attractive or rich enough to find a husband with more education, income, or job status than their own education potentially signified.

I've often thought, "How can I say my husband's a blue-collar repairman with less education than me when I worked my way through six years of college at night and full-time typing all day, working so hard for so long to get the graduate degree and make it as an author? At parties being an entrepreneur, an independent contractor means being employed. When saying I write full time, the answer I receive most often is, "Is that all you do?" or "Oh, so you're unemployed and don't earn a steady income." After my husband retired, I simply say, "He's retired." That's the great equalizer in social situations, like wearing a head-to-toe covering. Being a retiree equalizes the person with a graduate degree to the same playing field as the person who left college for feeling too old to compete.

The problem is solved. He's retired. My son and daughter reached forty-plus, and I've reached my mid-to-late-sixties. My son, the doctor is fine with his wife and children, all devout Muslims. I go to the synagogue when I need to and attend the Religious Science churches when I want to celebrate the celebration of life for all peoples in all worlds.

At the height of my career, being at the back end of sixty-something also is a great equalizer. The veil of invisibility descended just as surely as a burka or djellaba, with only a window to see out of behind the veil's grid of age-related eye floaters and flashes.

Suddenly I've rushed way past sixty-five, and no one wants to visit or hire me. So I just do the work without worrying whether I'm hired or not. I've hired myself. If the dream is big enough, the facts don't matter. If you know you have choices, the values in the choices outweigh the facts. It is now the time of reading, viewing, and listening to mind-body-spirit videos and recordings. It's the time for healing music. So I bought music composing software and returned to the music lessons that I halted in high school.

Something is greater out there than core identity. Whatever it is, it can include meditation and the chants of Tibetan monks. I paint Mandalas of deep archetypes as I write about serenity, harmony, and developing creativity while enhancing intuition in all areas of life, work, and play. Whether you write about relationships, finance, or machines, keep writing with great joy. Life is about personal broadcasting networks. Link all people to the one universal whole. That's where true happiness can be found.

I know how to paint 'wombs' in men—caverns of deep, physical thinking. A course in critical thinking taught me skepticism. But critical thinking and physical thinking are different. Logic hasn't evolved far enough beyond the cave to be critical. Not until rationality reaches and controls the stars (nature, space, and time) will it be able to fully evolve from the cave.

So there really doesn't have to be a schlemiel and a schlemazel—opposites, after all. Who needs polarity when you can experience irony by observing? You can seek joy of life through metaphor. You can seek visual anthropology through journalism.

Why be abstract when you can be concrete and write through and with the senses—including the sixth sense of intuition? You can view life up close or remotely from an armchair. Why view when you can have insight, hindsight, and foresight? Why observe as a journalist, when you can read how to avoid the pitfalls from anthropologists—my role models?

You can reach the universal through the details. The person is the archetype, and the archetype is the person. The universal abstract is in the concrete reality. The future is in the present. The person who is shy isn't really shy. He's only taking a sudden interest in his toes. That's the vignette within this novel. It's all about living the design-driven life. And the design-driven life has a purpose: To inspire and motivate persistence.

◆   ◆   ◆

23

Numerology and Marriage

One day in the present year I heard a media broadcast about numerology and how everyone is born with a particular 'tone' that can be expressed mathematically. Not only had I been told by astrologers doing a compatibility chart that I'd have trouble in my marriage because my 'Mars' was 'square' to my spouse's 'Mars,' but now numerology revealed my numerology number '8' when matched with my spouse's numerology '7' as mates were 'toxic to each other, with the number '7' husband undermining the number '8' wife's health.

After more than 32 years of marriage, numerology told me why I felt so ill, so off-center, and so unsafe when my mate came into the room or the rare times we went out together. The last time we were in a restaurant he said, "Are you going to eat all that food on your plate. You put too much food on that plate." Never had I felt so hungry for those few vegetables on my plate. At 120 pounds, five-feet four inches tall, why did he begrudge me that food pleasure? There weren't even any sweets on the plate. After 32+ years of a celibate marriage, why did I feel so denied?

Could it be because of my number eight in numerology and his number seven being toxic to each other? Or some other reason why I felt so unsafe and jittery around him and so joyous alone? Each time we had gone out to eat, walk, or listen to a lecture, he had made me cry. When alone I could be the real me and wander through little shops with art galleries or listen to healing music and let go of any stress. I had to find out why numerology told me so much, but still could apply to anyone's desire for financial security, love, and spirituality. I'd already been through the astrology conferences three decades before when astrologers told me that his chart said that he could do nothing for me. I married him anyway. Now numerology had to be explored as one more way people sought to look for patterns in nature and in mathematics.

Numerology is about the 'hidden' meaning of numbers and letters. Numerology is used to show differences of thinking between people. Humans look for patterns in statistical analysis or other mathematical symbols and also in nature that can be interpreted and applied to how one person affects another person's well-being, happiness, and stress levels.

By looking at my life destiny number (in numerology), it turns out I'm a number 'eight.' That is interpreted by numerology as having a need to seek happiness by finding financial security, managing my finances, and making money—the entrepreneurial sign. On the other hand, my spouse is a number 'seven,' the spiritual type who doesn't always want to talk or communicate verbally to a spouse. He's at home with every stranger, but a stranger in his own home so to speak. In other words, the individual can be extroverted with neighbors and introverted in the home with the wife. In the 32+ years of our marriage, I don't think we've talked more than five minutes before he blurts, "I'm outta here."

Now my number 8 (need to find financial security to be happy) birth path is softened by a destiny number 6 (creativity in writing or art and to be looked at by the public as having arrived at the top of my career and also be the nurturer, comforter, and healer), and my number 3 "inner guidance" wants communication, but my golden goal, a number 5 (travel and drama) wants to watch all those travel videos since I don't have any money to travel. Number 6 also signifies domesticity. And number 8 also signifies musicianship.

Ultimately the karmic lessons, which are the numbers missing in my name are 2 (love and peace in the home); 7 (spirituality) and 8, (finding and keeping what would make me happy—financial security and peace and love in the home above all.) But being married to a very frugal, thrifty and spiritual, but not religious number 7 is toxic to the number 8, but won't make any difference to the number 7. But what I really want is just pretty good health.

In other words, my astrological chart has the same interpretation as my numerology analysis. So I thought, if astrology is bunk and numerology is so accurate for me, would the analysis also apply to most people? Is my marriage toxic to me? It feels that way at my gut level, but not to my spouse. And is my need for financial security so deep rooted that there's no way I can simply walk out? Of course, logic says that as an older woman without more than a pittance of money of my own which would disappear in less than a year of lower middle class rental living, without insurance, friends, a place to go to, and completely alone would not be very happy either if I did simply walk out. So where do I go from here?

Probably back to being my number eight which says I'm destined to succeed and make a lot of money. But if I haven't made any money now that I'm well over 65 and not very mobile as a nondriver and rapidly aging by the day, where is this money coming from? Certainly my astrology chart predicts I'll never inherit any money from older relatives because there aren't older relatives, or if I've missed one or two, their money is destined for their own children and grandchildren, not me, of course. I wouldn't even know their last names. So how do I earn this money I'm destined to have by my numerology analysis? All I can do is write one book after another.

Just in case the reader wants to open a numerology business, the number 8 entrepreneur in me gives this helpful advice on how to start and run a numerology business at home or online. My creative number 6 versatility points to creating a video or audio podcast online about numerology. If you read enough books on exploring numerology and talk to practicing numerologists or take a course or seminar in numerology, it may open doors to becoming aware of any hidden meanings in numbers, letters, or even names.

Two books that helped me learn more about the subject that I highly recommend are: Exploring Numerology: Life By The Numbers, by Shirley Lawrence, New Page Books, Career Press, NJ 2003, and The Secret Science of Numerology: The Hidden Meaning of Numbers and Letters, also by Shirley Blackwell Lawrence, Msc.D. The book introduces the "Inner Guidance Number."

I enjoy reading on these topics, but the rational thinking course I've taken tells me to be careful not to be overtaken by my hunger for magical thinking as a way of solving problems I need to solve by step-by-step rational, skeptical thinking. On the other hand, I find prayer a form of "magical thinking" that turns on the spontaneous healing mechanism in my brain. What all these philosophies give me are more tools for healing by offering hope.

One example would be healing with harp and string music. Some people tell me hope is an excuse for not taking action through a specific behavior, that hope is an excuse for doing nothing. Other people say once you have hope, the spontaneous healing device in your brain gets turned on and certain defective genes can be switched on or off depending upon how deep your faith or hope is that you will be healed by the vibration of the music.

Is it all placebo effect, or is it all about using biofeedback to condition your brain and body to heal faster? I am free to try the simple solutions to happiness—mild Yoga, Tai Chi, Qi Gong, and healing music. I can read about Tibetan Buddhism or any other spiritual approach to natural healing. And I also can supplement with cutting out the sugar in my diet that's worsening my gum disease by raising my blood's glucose level so the anaerobic bacteria under the gum multiplies.

Is numerology science? Is astrology for real? If not, then why do so many leading military generals and commanders have a prominent 'Aries" in their astrology charts, and why does the astrological sign, 'Aries' signify military or war themes? The planets have nothing to do with us. The Greek/Roman deities are all man-made. So why are the charts so accurate when you put in the rising signs? Why does astrology say that my "secret enemy" is the person whose 'sun' sign is the same as my 'rising' sign on my "first house of health"?

In any case, speaking of numerology, which seems to agree with my astrology chart, what does it all mean? Why did numerology tell me exactly what my life has been like financially? Or is this all man-made to try and interpret nature? Is the real logic about looking at all this as magical thinking in the same way as pre-historic peoples tried to see patterns in nature and apply those patterns to understanding nature or healing?

If numerology interests you, then here's how to begin reading about starting and operating your own numerology business. You can follow a similar path to study any of the other 'noetic' arts from astrology to studying the symbolism of letters.

The noetic arts expand science beyond conventional paradigms. According to the Institute of Noetric Sciences, online at: http://www.noetic.org/, Noetic arts research potentials and powers of consciousness—including perceptions, beliefs, attention, intention, and intuition. Noetics explore phenomena not fitting into conventional scientific models, while maintaining a commitment to scientific rigor. Noetic arts view open-minded approaches on social and scientific topics. There are many ways of knowing.

Take the letter 'A' for example in several alphabets. In Hebrew and Phoenician, the letter A starts out as Aleph. In Greek, the letter 'A' is Alpha. Somewhere in time Aleph and Alpha once had a linguistic connection even though Alpha is Indo-European and Aleph is Semitic regarding the letter's linguistic classification. In Latin and English, the letter 'A' represents the first letter of the alphabet. Alpha or Aleph sounds similar because the Greek lettering system is based on the earlier Phoenician system.

In Biblical times, Aleph, the first letter of these alphabets mentioned above, received a label of being God's breath because you have to breathe out when you pronounce 'Aleph' (Ahhhhleff.). Since ancient humans needed to understand nature, you had to breathe out Aleph first, of course, before you could breathe out the next letter of those alphabets—Beth in Hebrew and Phoenician or Beta in Greek (and eventually B in Latin and English). When astrology developed, the letter A (Aleph) in Biblical times received the label of 'air.' Breath is air. Then

Aleph or Alpha in Levantine culture became associated with creation and the symbol of the 'Mother.'

Aleph is associated with the first breath a baby takes after being born. However, Aleph doesn't show up in astrology as an air sign. Instead it is an earth sign because in Hebrew and Phoenician the word, aleph, means ox head.

So the ox became the astrological sign of Taurus, associated with the shape of a uterus and all that is connected with giving birth, reproduction, and the breath that gives life. Interestingly, the astrology sign, Taurus started out representing female reproduction and ended up being represented by a male symbol, the bull, when it really represented the head of an ox. But when it's viewed in the night sky, it looks like a uterus with the ovaries and fallopian tubes moving upwards to form the ox's horns, according to the book titled, *The Secret Science of Numerology: The Hidden Meaning of Numbers and Letters*, by Shirley Blackwell Lawrence, Msc.D. New Page Books/Career Press, 2001.

It all boils down to people looking at the sky in ancient times to seek out patterns in order to understand and control nature. So how does all this become part of numerology used when trying to find a compatible mate? As a number 8, the entrepreneur, I see a small business for others in this pattern, and here's how to start and operate that business by beginning to learn how to do numerology readings, at least for entertainment only at parties, fundraisers, or in bookstores.

For example, suppose you enjoy new-age businesses, but you have no psychic abilities. Numerology and astrology rely on looking up information already written in books from ancient times to the present. So do businesses that tell you the hidden secrets or ancient philosophies regarding names and relationships or hidden markets for entrepreneurs.

On a certificated level, you can go to graduate school to become a licensed music or art therapist, and work in the healing fields using creative instruments and tools. But for those who want to teach themselves, you don't need a license to entertain with numerology. Here's how to begin learning about the subject and eventually run your own podcast or other online noetic arts-related business for entertainment.

You can sit in new-age or mind-body-spirit bookstores and give numerology readings or speak in public through online podcasting by audio or video as a small business or for entertaining, fundraising for charities, readings at alternative healing conventions and fairs, community center presentations, or at trade shows and expos.

Numerology Audio/Video Podcast Business for Entertaining and Fundraising

Numerologists interpret the numbers that determine life cycles and believe success is attracted to certain combinations of numbers. When you produce a numerology instructional video podcast, give clients readings by video podcast. Make sure that only the client can access the podcast on a Web site and download the reading. The podcast would only remain posted until the client has saved it.

As a numerologist, you give clients a reading based on how the client's first, middle, and last names influence their chances of success in finance, employment, marriage, or overall happiness. For entertainment purposes only, readings by numerologists, astrologists, or other practitioners work well with personal video podcasts that can be saved on iPods, mobile players, or in computers.

The videos can be saved to DVDs or CDs using compression software. Numerologists believe that you can change the way people react to you by changing your name, thereby influencing your chances for success.

Equipment Needed

You'll need your video podcasting software, a personal computer, video camcorder or digital video Web camera, DVD and CD recording drives, and disks. The estimated costs are about $1,000 worth of computer equipment and about $1,000-$3,000 for an industrial quality camcorder. Of course, you can use your digital high 8 camcorder, but the broadcast quality for professional-quality DVDs would be better with an industrial broadcast quality camcorder. For entertainment purposes, any digital video Web camera or amateur home video camcorder will record a reading.

Numerology software will be helpful. There is plenty of free numerology software on the Web for you to download. Some Web sites include: Decoz®Numerology—Free Numerology Software—Free Numerology Readings at: http://www.decoz.com/ and Numerology Software to purchase called Professional Numerologist at: http://www.wideninghorizons.com/. There is a free evaluation copy of numerology software to test before you buy. It's on the Web site at: http://www.wideninghorizons.com/download.shtml. A free Numerology Analysis Tool software is at: http://www.aboriginemundi.com/numerology.html. Search under "Numerology Software" as key words in your search engine online and find all types of numerology software, either free ware, evaluation copies, or software to purchase.

Operating Your New Age Numerology Video Podcast Business

To give a numerological reading, begin by obtaining the first, middle, and last name of your client and your client's birth date. In most interpretations of numerology each letter of the alphabet is assigned a number. These numbers are attributed with descriptions of personality. The numbers correspond to the following designations of the alphabet.

A B	C	D	E		F G	H I	J K	L M	N	O		P Q	R S	T U	V		W	X Y	Z
1 2	3	4	5		6 7	8 9	1 2	3 4	5	6		7 8	9 1	2 3	4		5	6 7	8

Number
1) leadership
2) artistic ability
3) humor
4) logical thinking
5) communications ability
6) domesticity
7) analytical and intellectual skills
8) business ethicality
9) entertainment

Some systems of numerology attribute personality quality to numbers. Number 9 in some systems is negative. By changing your name you avoid the repelling quality of your number.

In order to forecast with a numerological reading, you must add up the day, month, and year of a person's birth date and then add that figure to the sum arrived at from adding the letters of the first, middle, and last name. Then you take that sum and add the figures until you arrive at a number of 9 or less. For example, if you arrive at the number 22, each figure must be added until you get 4. The number 10 is 1 plus 0 or 1.

A person's reading consists of reducing all the numbers to between 1 and 9. One example is your client with the name "Anne Joan." These names are represented by the numbers 1555 and 1615. Add the numbers in the first name and the sum is 16. Add the two figures, and the sum is 7.

The next name adds up to 13. Then, 1 plus 3 equals 4. Take the 7 and 4 and add them to get 11. Add the 1 plus 1, and get a 2. Now take the number 2 and add it to the sum of the person's birth date. For example, if the person was born on November 18, 1941, it would be done this way: 1941 plus 11 plus 18. The sum total is 1970. Add each figure and get 17. Add these two figures to get one figure.

You end up with 8. Now add the number 2 from the name to 8 and get 10. Since one plus 0 is 1, your client is a number 1. In numerology number 1 means strong leadership ability. You could then advise your client to study for careers in which the leadership qualities would be used.

In addition to names, numerologists predict success is attracted to certain combinations of numbers in street addresses, telephone numbers, and other number sequences found in the life cycle that are believed to be predestined. Some numerologists predict stock market swings by observing recurring number cycles and ten-year patterns. Full instruction can be obtained by studying several good books on numerology and the instructions accompanying numerology software.

When you have learned the techniques, it's time to practice making private video podcasts of numerology readings for your clients. Your video podcasts also can be used to offer instruction and courses in numerology or related fields. In addition to numerology there are other 'noetic' areas to explore such as astrology or other types of readings.

Video podcasts work well when giving instruction in how to do numerology as most readings for clients are private and more suitable for saving on a CD or DVD. You wouldn't post private readings for clients on public Web sites, but you might put up a video for a client to download from a private site or send the client a CD or DVD with the video reading. The video podcast also may be produced in interview format.

Target Market

Convention attendees, party entertainment planners, public access TV panels, creative salons, interviewers, radio talk show hosts, community centers, senior centers, astrology and numerology clubs, and subscribers to numerology and/or astrology publications, students of numerology courses or subscribers related new-age, intuitive, and mind-body-spirit publications are all potential audiences. You can also write for niche newspapers and magazines, or attend new age fairs.

Other people in the mind-body-spirit arena include spiritualists, ministers of new age-related churches, mystic and noetic science course instructors, members of parapsychology clubs, and groups or publications interested in forecasting and insight may be interested. Even some nightclub acts may feature numerologists and mentalists.

Income Potential

For entertainment purposes, most numerologists on radio talk show are not paid. To give individual readings, a top-notch numerologist who is asked to speak on numerous radio or TV shows can ask for approximately $200 to answer a question or give a reading. Your purpose would be to help people figuratively balance.

Lesser known numerologists can ask anywhere from $15 to $25 or even $50 for a numerology reading. The more time you spend analyzing a client's numbers, the more you can ask. Readings also can be done online, by phone, or through video or audio podcasts. In video podcasting, the client can actually see how the numbers are grouped and interpreted if you have charts, Power point slide shows, or excellent quality video close-ups showing how you work with the numbers. How can podcasts work for you?

Don't forget other new age and health-related video podcast markets for exercises and workouts or touch and healing arts such as tai chi, qi gong, Reiki, and Yoga instruction and discussion. Research what 'Lightworkers' actually do. Can they be featured on video podcasts? Combine numerology with other venues.

Also check out the Web site for the Awakening Center at: http://www.theawakeningcenter.com/. Their site states, "OFALFO.org—a project of The Awakening Center, reaching out on the web and in the community, in Audio/Video/Text chats, community portal site and distance learning with a group of volunteers who give of their time and heart to assist others to find their 'center.' Continuing to grow and CO-create the essences for communicating in more vibrant methods to assist in reaching as many as we can."

An interesting quote from Phyllis Chesler's book titled *Woman's Inhumanity to Woman*, (Thunder's Mouth Press/Nation Books, New York, 2001, page 219, paragraph 3, line 5, reads, *"We never quite 'get over' or 'give up' our need for a Perfect Mother—some might say, for a loving God."*

What helped me most at any age emphasized reading more deeply into healing music, such as harp music and the use of the expressive and creative art therapies when combined with improved nutrition. I had to look at myself from the genes, that molecular level upwards. What finally calmed the panic disorder and agoraphobia for me focused on walking and stretching away agoraphobia and panic disorder with Tai Chi, Qi Gong, and gentle Yoga. Balance became the focus. Nutrition came first.

Gentle bellydancing helped me slowly stretch to the healing music. Ultimately, a moderate walking and stretching exercise and nutrition program helped me along with the nutrition change. This book is meant to inspire you to help yourself as much as you can with what works well for you as an individual.

Do the best with what you have. It's wise to see yourself as a series of connections, a whole person, in the mind-body-spirit sense and not only as a symptom. Becoming aware of how you are connected is the first step. That's what you can do as you work along with your health care professionals—become aware of how you are connected from the molecular level on upwards and how your genes affect your own behavior, body, and mind. Find out why humans seek to understand themselves and nature by seeking patterns in every connection. Then look at the statistics in the various tests. Which patterns recur many times in significant ways? What do these patterns mean to you?

Bibliography

Freedom From Agoraphobia by Mark Eisenstadt, M.D. (December 2003)

Master Your Panic and Take Back Your Life: Twelve Treatment Sessions to Conquer Panic, Anxiety and Agoraphobia, _ by Denise F. Beckfield. Nov. 2003.

The Agoraphobia Workbook: A Comprehensive Program to End Your Fear of Symptom Attacks by C. Alec Pollard and Elke Zuercher-White (Jun 2003)

Change Your Brain, Change Your Life: The Breakthrough Program for Conquering Anxiety, Depression, Obsessiveness, Anger, and Impulsiveness, by Daniel G. Amen. Dec 31, 1999.

Overcoming Panic Disorder and Agoraphobia: Client Manual (Best Practices for Therapy Series) by Elke Zuercher-White. May 1999.

Life Isn't Just a Panic: Stories of Hope by Recovering Agoraphobics by Anita L. Pace. 1996.

When Bad Genes Happen to Good People by Nesse, RM. Technology Review. May/June 1995, ppg 31-40.

Treatment Of Panic Disorder With And Without Agoraphobia: January 1985 Through July 1991 : 1448 Citations, by Karen Patrias; Barry Wolfe; National Library of Medicine (U.S.). Reference Section. Publisher: Bethesda, Md. U.S. Dept. of Health and Human Services, Public Health Service, National Institutes of Health, National Library of Medicine, Reference Section ; Washington, D.C. : Supt. of Docs., U.S. G.P.O.

Hope and Help for Your Nerves (Signet) by Claire Weekes. 1990.

Predictive Medicine for Rookies: Consumer Watchdogs, Reviews, & Genetics Testing Firms Online, by Anne Hart. Apr 2005.

How to Write Plays, Monologues, or Skits from Life Stories, Social Issues, or Current Events: For All Ages, by Anne Hart. May 2004.

Murder in the Women's Studies Department: A Professor Sleuth Novel of Mystery, by Anne Hart. Mar. 2002.

Writing 7-Minute Inspirational Life Experience Vignettes: Create and Link 1,500-Word True Stories, by Anne Hart. June 2004.

How to Refresh Your Memory by Writing Salable Memoirs with Laughing Walls: A Pop-Culture Course in Reminiscing for Pay, by Anne Hart. Oct. 2006.

Employment Personality Tests Decoded, by Anne Hart with George Sheldon. Career Press. July 2007.

The Cult of Personality, by Annie Murphy Paul, Free Press. 2004.

◆   ◆   ◆

Index

978-0-595-43402-2
0-595-43402-9

www.ingramcontent.com/pod-product-compliance
Lightning Source LLC
Chambersburg PA
CBHW030314290526
45785CB00001B/349